# Faculty Practice Plans

*Models for a New Health Care Age*

Edited by James E. Casanova, MD

**AMERICAN COLLEGE OF PHYSICIAN EXECUTIVES**
4890 West Kennedy Boulevard, Suite 200
Tampa, Florida 33609-2575
813/287-2000

# Table of Contents

**Chapter 1**    Introduction ........................................................................1
*by James E. Casanova, MD*

**Chapter 2**    An Overview of the Critical Elements
in a Faculty Practice Plan ..................................................5
*by John Bernard Henry, MD, FACPE*

**Chapter 3**    Managed Care and Health Care Market Reform ....................13
*by Martin E. Hickey, MD, MS, FACPE*

**Chapter 4**    Teaching in the Faculty Practice Setting ...............................23
*by Mark Kushner, MD, Shari L. Bornstein, MD, MPH,
and Roger Hand, MD*

**Chapter 5**    Faculty Practice Plan Governance and Management ............33
*by William H. Frishman, MD*

**Chapter 6**    The Faculty Practice Plan in a Public Teaching Hospital.......37
*by William L. Boddie, MD*

**Chapter 7**    Department Practice Plan to Respond
to Managed Care Environment.................................................43
*by Gene F. Conway, MD, John Dorfmeister, MA,
and Robert G. Luke, MD*

**Chapter 8**    Establishing a Centralized Faculty Practice Plan...................53
*by Martin S. Litwin, MD*

**Chapter 9**    Mixed Faculty Practice Plan Model in Transition .................67
*by Paul H. Rockey, MD, MPH*

**Chapter 10**    Practice Plan Associates: A Plan in Transition........................77
*by Joel A. Kaplan, MD, and Milton H. Sisselman, MS*

**Chapter 11**    Centralization Key Goal of Faculty Practice Plan.................85
*by Rein Saral, MD, and Garland D. Perdue, MD*

**Chapter 12**　　Pediatrics Faculty Practice Plan Looks
to Managed Care Future ..........................................................93
*by James A. Menke, MD, Richard E. McClead, MD,
and Mitchell Wheller, BS, MHA*

**Chapter 13**　　Centralization Characterizes University of Arkansas Plan.....99
*by F. Patrick Maloney, MD, MPH*

**Chapter 14**　　A Faculty Practice Plan within a Community/
University Integrated Medical Education Program ....................109
*by Tom M. Johnson, MD, FACP, and John L. Jones Jr., MA, MBA*

# Chapter 1

▲  ▲  ▲

## Introduction

by James E. Casanova, MD

When this book was first conceived, more than four years ago, academic health centers, like the health care delivery system overall, were in a state of turmoil. They were caught in the frenzy of change that has characterized organizational health care for most of the past decade. The frenzy and turmoil continue. Managed care has moved, not very quietly, from a major role in the delivery and financing of health care services to a starring role. Its penetration in many markets exceeds the 50 percent level, and more than one-third of all Americans now receive their health care through managed care plans. Employers report that nearly 80 percent of all employees are covered by managed care plans. Most observers expect the domination of managed care to continue and grow.

More important than these numbers, however, is the extent to which managed care and its offspring have transformed the business of health care. The key word is "competition." And competition in health care is increasingly based on and fed by contractual delivery of services to defined populations of consumers—patients. Free movement of patients within the health care delivery system is nearly a thing of the past. In most health maintenance organization approaches to care, such movement is not possible, or is possible only with the permission of the HMO. In other forms of managed care, preferred provider organizations and their brethren, movement is restricted or carries a higher price tag for the patient. Success in this competitive environment requires packaging potential users of health care services in contractual arrangements, developing owned and contracted organizations to provide promised services, and instituting controls that ensure that services are provided in a rational and cost-effective manner.

Academic health centers have been slow to respond to these new forces. The high technical levels of care that are taken for granted in this country will require that academia continue to serve as the main staging area for research on disease and injury and on how they will be treated and cured. Research activities will have to be largely funded from outside the health care delivery system. The teaching mission must also continue unabated if we expect to have practitioners who can use the results of research to the benefit of patients. Of course, academic health centers will have to improve their record in introducing tomorrow's clinicians to managed care and all the other structural changes in how health care is delivered and financed. But it is difficult to see how they can respond to cost issues in the same way that other provider organizations can. Academic medicine, by its very nature, is more expensive.

It is in the third mission of the academic health center, however, that the greatest impact of managed care and other structural and financial changes has been felt. Academic health centers are major providers of patient care. Their research and teaching depend on a steady stream of patients presenting diseases and injuries that instruct the student and inspire the teacher and researcher. Further, the income from patient care activities has been a major source of funding for teaching and research. The three missions are a package, and damage to any one of them bodes ill for survival of the academic health center. But, as already stated, research and teaching are expensive, and demands for patient care income are high. The managed care approach is intended to squeeze patient care income, and this places academic health centers at a competitive disadvantage.

For several decades now, patient care activities in academic health centers have been organized around faculty practice plans, dominated, as have been academic health centers generally, by medical specialists. Of course, specialists have dominated financial aspects of health care delivery throughout the health care system. But managed care is changing the relationship between primary care physicians and specialists, and those changes are now visiting academia. Controlling the costs of care requires reevaluation of the definition of "best care," of the roles of specialists and generalists, and of the systems in which they practice medicine.

## Purpose of This Book
And that brings us to the purpose of this book. How are faculty practice plans responding to the changes that surround them? In the following chapters, leaders in the academic health care field discuss in detail the changes that are occurring in academic health care delivery. Chapters 2-4 discuss academic health care delivery in generic terms, providing a background for the final ten chapters, case studies of faculty practice plans that have made the transition to a managed care, competitive world. Our goal has been to provide some road maps, complete with warning signs, that will allow physicians in academic settings to plot a course through the jungle of change that lies ahead.

## Background and Issues
In Chapter 2, Dr. John Bernard Henry puts the faculty practice plan in perspective, describing the gridwork on which faculty practice plans operate, now and in the future. There are essential elements in a faculty practice plan, regardless of the environment in which it operates or the forces with which it must deal. The particulars of these elements will vary from plan to plan and from institution to institution, but all of them will have to be analyzed and reconstructed as faculty practice plans redefine themselves. As Dr. Henry emphasizes, faculty practice plans must understand what they are and how they fulfill their current missions if they are to have any hope of competing or networking successfully with nonacademic health care organizations.

Dr. Martin Hickey lays out the full scope of the managed care world in Chapter 3, describing it in both general and academic health center terms. As they are currently structured, Dr. Hickey says, faculty practice plans have little hope of doing well in a managed care environment. And he cautions academia not to believe that managed care is merely a phase that can be safely ignored. The changes it will force are fundamental, and they will not be easy for organizations that are wary of change, slow in their reactions, and sometimes more attentive to themselves and their designated missions than to the publics they serve. But he points to several factors that make the motivated academic health center an ideal candidate for success in a managed care world.

In Chapter 4, Drs. Mark Kushner, Shari Bornstein, and Roger Hand describe the shift throughout the health care system to a primary care focus and offer strong evidence for the ability of academic health centers to respond successfully to this trend. In a series of case reports, they show how several academic health centers and faculty practice plans have combined an emphasis on research and education in primary care with successful models for delivery of primary care services. There are major difficulties with the teaching mission in faculty practices, they say, but they can be overcome. Creativity is the key, and they describe some creative responses that have already been made.

## The Case Reports

The ten case studies that conclude the book are not meant to be exhaustive. We believe, however, that they are both instructive and illuminating. Were there room, we could have included reports on all existing faculty practice plans. Our fear, well-founded we believe, was that the benefits of this extensive treatment would not have justified the size of the volume required for its presentation.

Our ten reports cover both private and public medical school systems. Both centralized and decentralized approaches are represented, although we think that the evidence supports a trend toward the centralization that earlier chapters predicted. The cases clearly show the impact of managed care. Faculty practice plans, as here represented, are grappling with managed care. The focus may be still be too much on physician income, but significant structural changes are being undertaken.

Our expectation was that the case studies would show substantial attention to the interface of academia and the remainder of the health care delivery and financing system. Our reading now is that academia is still essentially parochial in its views. Measures taken to-date, if the case reports are representative, have been defensive in nature, attempts to shore up faculty practice plans rather than prepare them for the full force of competition that surely awaits them. However, there are seeds in the centralized plans for successful entry on the competitive field.

And that leads to a final and critical point. In a time of frenzy and turmoil, it is wise to consider today's offerings merely prologue. Much lies ahead. Many of these case reports have undergone substantial changes during production of the book. As you read the book, they are likely undergoing further change. Our goal has been to show that change can be handled successfully. All of these faculty practice plans have assimilated the concept of change and are, we think, better prepared to deal with the future. What is important, and instructive, about the faculty practice plans presented in this book is the direction in which they are headed and the flexibility that they are building into their operations.

*James E. Casanova, MD, is Assistant Dean, Clinical Affairs, Medical College of Wisconsin, Milwaukee.*

# Chapter 2

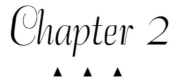

## An Overview of the Critical Elements
## in a Faculty Practice Plan

by John Bernard Henry, MD, FACPE

*A* faculty practice plan (FPP) serves the medical faculty within an academic department, division, or section committed to practicing medicine under the auspices of an academic health center or university whose mission includes education; research; patient care; and, often, community service. It also serves the health center and university through an increasing proportion of revenue and as a source of patients for education.[1] Organizationally, an FPP may be described primarily as institutional (centralized) or department-based (decentralized).[2] A medical service group (MSG) constitutes a department or clinical discipline of plan members and is, in turn, under the umbrella of the FPP and is a constituent with representation on the governing board of the FPP. Individual members may be classified as independent contractors, partners, or employees.

An FPP is a legal document that describes the rules, regulations, policies and procedures, and relationships among members and between the plan and others in the academic health center, especially administration. The academic health center and/or parent university establishes overriding guidelines through policies and procedures to which individual clinical departments, divisions, or sections in a decentralized FPP or centralized plan must adhere in generating their own bylaws, rules, regulations, and policies and procedures.

A governance structure is established for each FPP and MSG; these governing relationships in turn are described within the overall academic health center and/or university governing body, with the latter comprising university or academic health center leaders and managers. Mutual responsibility and authority with accountability are defined for each FPP and MSG and its governing body within the context of the university and academic health center operational management.

The purpose of this chapter is to provide an overview of the critical elements in a faculty practice plan (FPP), a complex entity with several constituencies within an academic health center and university organization. While there are about 40 freestanding academic health centers among the total of 127, most centers exist within private and public universities in terms of operations management and organization.[2] For these critical elements of each FPP, there is a variety of permutations that may be adapted or modified to meet the specific needs of the health center and university and of plan members, depending on culture, environment, personalities, priorities, and values within an academic health center; virtually all are currently experiencing transformation.

The central or essential critical elements of a FPP will nevertheless be identified and addressed insofar as possible to appreciate what must or should be in place to achieve success in an effective, efficient clinical practice with a sufficient margin of revenues over expenses in a collegial atmosphere to meet the needs of individual members and the university while pursuing the academic mission of education and research. After 35 to 40 years of existence, FPPs are in place for virtually all 127 academic health centers. While a new or startup FPP initiative is unlikely, the varied elements to be described must be in place for both new and existing plans.

## Culture, Philosophy, and Organization

*Culture* describes what permeates an organization in terms of human behavior, customs, and values. An understanding of the culture provides insight into the organization, especially in terms of priorities within the objectives of an FPP or an MSG.[3] An academic health center or university is the overall organization within which both decentralized (MSGs) or centralized (often medical school or medical center) faculty practice plans exist.

A *philosophy* of funding research and education through surplus patient care revenue may be observed. However, other philosophies exist, e.g., excellence in patient care service as a foundation for teaching and research. The philosophical relationships among the critical elements of education, research, and patient care should be identified in terms of emphasis or prioritization.

Among the elements that help one appreciate the *organization* are overall management, including policies and procedures for cost-effective and efficient billing for medical services provided by the clinical faculty through centralized billing and collection. Administrative or management support of an FPP, e.g., space allocation with or without assigned costs and adequate support staff, also need to be considered. The net contribution of a faculty practice plan to support of the academic health center, often identified with the "dean's tax" or other contributions to support education and research, should also be made clear to FPP members.

A faculty practice plan table of organization (TO) within an academic medical center is vital to identify the chain of command and the extent of faculty members' participation in decision making. A TO should identify MSG and FPP governance, i.e., governing board relation to the university and/or the academic medical center board of directors. Each MSG should have bylaws, rules, and regulations that have been endorsed by top administration and any appropriate governing boards.

Organizational features for private and public medical centers vary and to appreciate them as critical elements is important. Bentley and colleagues[2] noted in 1991 that private medical schools more often (74 percent) had FPPs within schools. In public schools, 57 percent of the plans were organized within the school and 43 percent were outside the school.

Departments, divisions, or associations within the medical school or university structure predominated (62 percent), while 38 percent were separate and independent legal entities. These legal entities include not-for-profit or for-profit corporations; foundations; charitable trusts; partnerships, including the more recently developed limited liability partnerships; and professional corporations (PCs), all are usually outside the university or institution.

A not-for-profit entity is exempt partially if not totally from federal, state, and local taxes. Private universities offer this advantage within the university to a FPP, most often in a centralized form but also in a decentralized form with MSGs.

The organizational structure of faculty practice plans is evolving from department-based MSGs to more centralized, integrated, multidisciplinary faculty practice plan entities. This transformation may be attributed to two forces. A multidisciplinary group practice is a more competitive entity to reckon with in private practice. It is also a single entity to establish contractual relations with HMOs or PPOs, insurance carriers; or other third-party payers in a competitive health care delivery environment of managed care. In other words, it makes the several separate medical services groups and clinical disciplines virtually a single entity, with a single voice type of decision making, i.e., more prompt. The integrated plans incorporate all of the clinical departments. Arrangement of the plan as a multidisciplinary group practice then permits identification of physicians and/or hospitals, including physician-hospital organizations (PHOs), as integrated inpatient and ambulatory care services with satellite, off-campus clinics with or without their own HMOs.[4] The more centralized, more efficient practice plans that join through their college of medicine with their teaching hospital will be the ones that will be least harmed by the economic changes that have developed and are developing. Identification of an ambulatory care facility and a centralized billing system with management support are hallmarks of a high degree of centralization of administration and management functions to facilitate practice.

## Governance
Certain overriding elements of governance exist within both the more organized centralized FPPs and the decentralized MSGs. First and foremost are the university's faculty practice plan guidelines, generated primarily by university administration with variable degrees of medical faculty input. Faculty members, who are generally chairs or other leaders, may, in conjunction with the dean and/or vice president of medical affairs and his or her chief financial officer, establish policy and overall guidelines for the FPP, usually through a governing board. This overall policy may also be accomplished through a university board of directors in conjunction with the university president.

An integrated governing board representing MSGs or a centralized plan as a distinct level of governance can show concordance within the university academic health center and its faculty. This reflects a good fit of a faculty practice plan with or within the university academic health center. In other words, it is a more comfortable interface between the faculty practice plan members and the university or administration. As an overall governing body, it is also a vehicle for strategic planning and plan changes, with accountability for budget and fiscal decisions and assurance of proper timely payments to the university or the academic medical center. The governing board receives, approves, and monitors individual medical service group budgets for expenses and revenues. The medical group fiscal and operational autonomy is respected but, at the same time, overall accountability of the university through a governing board is in place to sustain fiscal solvency. Representation on such a governing board is from appointed faculty; from department, section, or division chairs; and/or from elected faculty representatives.[5]

The board is key to negotiations for change in an FPP and the point at which different clinical disciplines, through their MSGs, may debate policy modifications. Such debate between clinical disciplines and between governing board and university, academic health center, or medical school administration, personified in the medical dean and/or the vice president of the center, can be contentious. This is especially true where "fiefdoms" and/or "big earners" with lucrative practices exist.[6]

Another important level of governance usually resides in a department, section, or division operating as an MSG, where harmony and shared values among clinical faculty members should be observed or promulgated but are not always observed. Here, faculty leaders, such as department chairs or division/section heads, oversee management operations in terms of the most efficient, cost-effective medical practice within the policies or guidelines of the university. This is also where further policies are defined and refined and faculty compensation and benefits evolve and are monitored. Fee schedules of departments, sections, and divisions of clinical faculty are also regularized in terms of equity and parity among medical service groups within the academic health center and comparable clinical disciplines outside the university. This is done very carefully and sensitively to avoid any hint of collusion or action that would invoke antitrust regulation review. Financial impact of Medicare fee schedules is assessed at this level of governance.[7]

The university administration and governing board validate accountability for FPP/MSG fund distributions. Open disclosure of finances in an FPP or MSG should provide information on the flow of funds and the margins of revenue over expenses (or deficits) for individual practice units through income and balance statements plus verbal presentations and discussions. Disclosure of financial information shows the faculty's confidence in and commitment to the plan, as well as loyalty to the university. When an FPP or an MSG experiences a deficit or begins to accumulate debt, the bells ring for action. Other MSGs or health center or university administration need to take appropriate action to avoid insolvency for the FPP or MSG and extension of the financial problems to the health center or university. This may be in the form of a loan or a temporary subsidy, but it may also require changes in the chair or the MSG leadership.

Revenue distribution among faculty practice plans is a challenging as well as sensitive subject and may be a source of tension among FPP participants through their individual chairs/departments as centralized or decentralized entities (MSGs) and university academic medical center administration; the administration is most often perceived as the medical school dean and/or Vice President of Medical Affairs who may also be a president in a freestanding academic health center. A compensation ceiling for faculty defined by university administration in academic health centers in terns of faculty rank and/or other responsibility is a critical issue to be addressed from the standpoint of faculty as well as administration. This may be more challenging in terms of salary plus benefits reflecting total compensation versus a salary ceiling alone. Likewise, the medical service group or FPP/MSG contributions to the university, whether it is a dean's tax or other assessments, need to be carefully addressed. Both compensation to faculty in medical service groups and medical service group contributions to the university may be negotiable in certain institutions to variable degrees.

A faculty practice plan must also include a *mission statement* that is based on the *philosophy* of the institution and a *policy and procedure* manual spelling out details of operations and relations among faculty members and between faculty members in MSGs and the university or academic health center. Good communication among the governing board, departments, and individual physicians is crucial in today's competitive, often tense, and constantly changing health care delivery environment.

## Faculty Salaries, Benefits, and Tenure

Faculty members today require competitive compensation that is in line with, if it does not approach or approximate, that of peer physicians in private practice, They are more like such practicing clinicians than more traditional academic physicians, with less time for research and education than their academic peers because of major practice commitments. FPP funding within the overall plan operations and assisting the medical school/center and its clinical or basic science departments are considered within the FPP/MSG contribution and commitment to university/ center.

Clinical faculty members heavily involved in practice compete with academic peers on a tenure tract. All faculty members are expected to teach, whether they are on a tenure or a nontenure tract. However, the amount or percentage of teaching varies among clinical disciplines and institutions. Hence, clinical tracts (nontenure) for faculty members have become more widespread in academia over the past decade. Is the faculty practice plan incentive-based, and how much entrepreneurism is supported and encouraged? These are important questions to consider under any conditions, but especially in the construction of a nontenure track.

Five-year-term, renewable contracts often are a critical element in appointment and reappointment for faculty on a nontenure or clinical track. This is in vivid contrast to the perception that tenured faculty have essentially "life-time" faculty appointments with the exception of fiscal exigency and/or abolishment of an academic program including faculty in place. For clinical track appointees, the notification date is usually one year in advance of the termination date, i.e., year 4 versus year 5. Also, the time interval (number of years) to faculty before appointment is terminated is most important. Because these usually are five-year term appointments on a clinical track, individual faculty members need to know whether or not they are going to be reappointed, and this notification is usually forthcoming a year in advance of the five-year concluding interval. In other words, faculty members need to make plans for relocating elsewhere and the university needs to notify individuals that their appointments will not be continued beyond specific dates. This is an element of insecurity and concern among clinical track appointees that needs to be appreciated and addressed in a timely manner. Hence the notification date and time interval to faculty before appointment is terminated or renewed should be incorporated into contractual relations of employee, independent contractor, and partner members.

Compensation includes salary and all fringe benefits and takes into account individual FPP members' practice expenses. This broad definition allows creative compensation arrangements, so salary and benefits should be carefully delineated both individually and collectively. This delineation is especially important if benchmark targets serve as the compensation reference for a medical school, e.g., a goal of 80 percent of the Association of American Medical Colleges' national compensation levels for each discipline or a university salary schedule for each faculty rank.

Among clinical practice disciplines are the "have nots," e.g., pediatrics, and the "haves", e.g., surgery. These and other perceived imbalances among clinical faculty practices in terms of revenue, expense, and net income warrant careful consideration and mutual understanding. Revenue-generation and compensation disparities exist and must be managed carefully and sensitively.[8,9]

Faculty members perceive the money they generate as belonging to them. This perception may or may not be shared by the health center and university administration. Hence, these aspects of compensation can be a contentious element unless clarified at initial appointment. Priorities in expenses and in revenue allocations must be accomplished in a manner that accords respect to high income generators and equity in their contributions or in redistribution of FPP revenue to other university departments through the university administration. Indeed, FPP or MSG assessment/contribution to the university or medical center, i.e., percentage of gross or net FPP revenue, may become critical elements. "Fiefdom" thinking and behavior are common in an environment of competition and managed care and are a challenge for leadership at all levels. Faculty cohesiveness and commitment to a unified multidisciplinary group practice, while supporting the overall academic enterprise, will ensure survival in the '90s and into the next century.

## Trust and Respect

Ultimately, mutual trust and respect among faculty members and their department leadership and university or academic health center administration are crucial. The establishment of trust and respect is related to good communication, mutual support, responsiveness to the needs of faculty members, and faculty efficiency in terms of practice, education, and research. Nurturance of faculty creativity requires a measure of autonomy for faculty members expected to both practice and teach. It also requires leadership and fine-tuned, sensitive management at all levels of the organization. Innovative faculty and organizational leadership are most important in a competitive health care delivery system to manage the stress academic health centers (faculty and administration) are experiencing in a changing environment. A large measure of the stress reflects greater university dependence on FPP revenues because of pressures on medical school tuition revenue, less well-supported research, and diminishing university or public (state and federal) funding. Faculty members may have less time to devote to research and thus remain competitive for grant funding and less time to teach because of increased patient care services.

## Summary

FPPs have functioned for more than 40 years, to the point that virtually all academic health centers and medical schools have them. Their evolution over the years has not been without friction and major accommodation by faculty members and administration. With the changes in academic medicine and the increasingly competitive health care delivery system, the evolution will surely continue. An appreciation of the critical elements in an FPP should be helpful in the transformation. Collegiality and cooperation among faculty and between clinical disciplines and administration are vital to this evolution.

## References

1. Jones, R., and Sanderson, S. "Clinical Revenues Used to Support the Academic Mission of Medical Schools." *Academic Medicine* 71(3):299-307, March 1996.

2. Bentley, J., and others. "Faculty Practice Plans: the Organization and Characteristics of Academic Medical Practice." *Academic Medicine* 66(8): 433-9, Aug. 1991.

3. MacLeod, G., and others. "An Attitudinal Assessment of Faculty Practice Plans." *JAMA* 257(8):1072-5, Feb. 27, 1987.

4. Culbertson, R. "How Successfully Can Academic Faculty Practices Compete in Developing Managed Care Markets?" *Academic Medicine* 71(8):858-70, Aug. 1996.

5. Bunch, W., and Siegler, A. "What Faculty Members Value in Practice Plans." *Journal of Medical Education* 62(10):799-804, Oct. 1987.

6. Wilczek, K. "The Evolution of Faculty Practice Plans." *Topics in Health Care Financing* 16(3):83-7, Spring 1990.

7. Billi, J., and others. "Financial Impact of the Medicare Fee Schedule on a Large Multispecialty Faculty Practice in an Academic Medical Center." *Academic Medicine* 68(5):315-22, May 1993.

8. Karp, R. "University Surgical Group." *Annals of Thoracic Surgery* 60(5):1481-5, Nov. 1995.

9. Lewis, J. "Improving Productivity: the Ongoing Experience of an Academic Department of Medicine." *Academic Medicine* 71(4):317-28, April 1996.

*John Bernard Henry, MD, FACPE, is Professor, Department of Pathology, College of Medicine, and Director of Transfusion Medicine, Histocompatibility, Stem Cell, and Parentage Laboratories, University Hospital, SUNY Health Science Center at Syracuse, Syracuse, New York. Dr. Henry is Past President of the Health Science Center.*

# Chapter 3

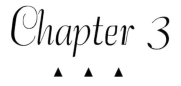

## Managed Care and Health Care Market Reform

by Martin E. Hickey, MD, MS, FACPE

## Introduction

The impact of managed care on academic medicine will be no less than that of the Flexner report on medical education. Academic medicine and its accompanying medical centers evolved and flourished in an era of unlimited fee-for-service reimbursement. Not only did their financing mechanisms become highly dependent on this payment method, but much of their political and value structures developed around it as well. The three-legged stool of research, education, and patient care is being transformed by managed care into a tricycle, with the front wheel (which has the pedals) being patient care. The rider is no longer the Chief of Surgery, but rather the Chief of Family Medicine! The adaptation of academic medicine, academic medical centers, and faculty practice plans to the new managed care environment will require the dismantling of the stool as we have come to know it. In turn, managed care will require the design and construction of an agile and extremely fast vehicle, powered by primary care and steered by a centralized leadership to outmaneuver and outrun the community competition.

## Why Managed Care?

Because American medicine has apparently been so successful in its pursuit of scientific quality, the center of which activity has been in academic medicine, most medical faculty members cannot understand the rapid migration of patients from academic medical centers to health maintenance organizations (HMOs). But managed care would not exist unless there was a real societal need, and that need is for value. Value can be defined as the quality of a product or service, the customer orientation with which it is delivered, and the cost required to produce it. Most academic faculty members would contend that health care is a virtually unmeasurable service that has such intrinsic value in and of itself that business definitions cannot be assigned to it. Further, the pursuit of scientific medical knowledge through research is also a stand-alone virtue that should be pursued irrespective of cost.

But academic medical faculty members do not pay for health care services. Employers, which have to compete in a highly competitive world market, and government, which has to tame an out-of-control budget deficit, have determined that the cost has become far too high. Costs reached more than a trillion dollars and 14 percent of the Gross Domestic Product in 1995, and increases in health care have routinely been two to three times general inflation over the past several years. These economic conditions have created a rapid and relentless surge to managed care from coast to coast.

The high cost of health care can be attributed to a multiplicity of factors, including technology advancement, increasing enfranchisement of the poor and elderly through government programs, expanded coverage of benefits from employers, increased demand for services on the part of patients, the increasing number of specialists, and so on. But the critical feature that enabled health care cost increases to occur has been the structure of financial reimbursement created by fee-for-service indemnity insurance. Through this financing mechanism, the patient has come to expect full and uninhibited care and to pay little or nothing for it. Under fee-for-service financing, physicians and hospitals have been able to raise prices unchecked to cover costs, produce desired operating margins, and maintain incomes (which, for physicians, averaged a 10 percent annual increase during the 1980s). Insurers readily paid the charges and passed the annual 10-25 percent increases to employers in the next year's premium.

Managed care has been a response from employers to control their health insurance premium costs when no other mechanism existed for this purpose. The evolution of managed care companies, or health plans, is nothing more than the creation of the classic American "middle man" to serve a purpose that the user (employers) and producers (physicians and hospitals) couldn't or wouldn't undertake themselves. Now managed care has a life and rationale of its own and will dominate health care delivery as long as it can continue to produce value for payer.

## Essential Features of Managed Care

There are six essential components to the current evolution of managed care:

▲ Capitation—prepaid health care delivery via per member per month payments.

▲ Primary Care—organization of care through generalist providers.

▲ Data—dependence of quality and cost of care on information feedback.

▲ Systems—organizational requirement for the development and feedback of data and incentive alignment to contain costs.

▲ Competition—purchase of health care services through systems on the basis of value comparisons.

▲ Value—the ability of a system to provide low cost, high outcome quality, and outstanding "customer" service.

### Capitation

Initial efforts to contain costs via managed care programs were only incrementally successful, primarily because providers and health care institutions could usually game rules and incentives established to contain costs. Cost is a factor of price, volume, and intensity. Initial managed care plans focused on controlling price by discounts, a set fee schedule, and/or a percentage withhold of reimbursement (returned at the end of the fiscal year if prospective allocation targets were met). But what was lost in price by a provider could easily be recovered in volume. If volume was tracked and determined to be excessive by a health plan, the provider could recover losses by increasing the intensity of services.

The most efficient method of ending the gaming and the need for expensive policing of the provider is to pass the risk for resource utilization from the plan to the provider. The easiest way to accomplish this is to prospectively pay the provider (primary care clinician, specialist, and hospital) on a monthly basis for each member of the managed care plan designated to receive care from that provider. This is what capitation, a per member per month payment (pmpm), does. Thus, price per visit or procedure, volume, and intensity of resources brought to bear by the provider become irrelevant. The provider now has the incentive to not overutilize resources or not add unnecessary volume. Also, who could better make the judgment of what resources to utilize than the provider, who, with good data feedback, has the medical and economic knowledge to utilize resources appropriately. Physicians, through their pens, control about 80 percent of all health care costs. If the physician does not write the order, the care cannot take place. If the physician, by retaining the unspent prospective capitation payment, has an incentive not to overutilize, costs will be significantly contained through the physician's pen.

There are important quality and ethical issues raised by this turn to prospective payment and provider risk assumption. In time, these issues will have to be addressed as competition moves beyond cost and is based more on quality and service. But as a method of containing costs, the central issue of the current health care reform debate, the approach is extremely successful. After one to two decades of double-digit medical inflation, capitation not only has succeeded in containing costs in California and other pockets in the West, but also has actually reversed the cost of care; that is, there is medical deflation! As providers have assumed risk for their own practice patterns, and especially for hospital and specialty utilization, resource utilization has plummeted through the elimination of unnecessary care. For example, length of stay averages for 1,000 commercial health plan members have dropped from more than 600 days in the late eighties to less than 150 in many Western health plans employing capitation. These savings are being passed to purchasers in the form of lower premiums.

### Primary Care
The move to capitation has added significant value to the role of the primary care provider. Who better to designate as the coordinator and center of care. A primary care physician— family practitioner; general internist; pediatrician; and, in some plans, obstetrician—has the ability to provide most routine care and has the knowledge base to pass responsibility for care to a specialist when indicated. The primary care clinician should also have the capability, or can be trained to have the capability, to take back the management of patients with relatively stable chronic diseases. Further, when in financial alignment with a managed care plan and when given appropriate data on costs and outcomes, the general practitioner can act as a successful purchasing and monitoring agent on behalf of the plan and the patient for provision of the most efficient and effective hospital and specialist care.

Aside from these important roles in a managed care delivery system, the primary care practitioner has significantly increased value because there are so few of them. Even if all residencies turned out 50 percent primary care physicians starting in 1995, it would take until 2040 to achieve a national 50 percent generalist balance.

## Data

Primary care clinicians cannot monitor the efficiency and effectiveness of their own and others' care without good data on the cost and outcomes of care. The same is true for specialists, hospitals, and health plans. It is particularly critical to have data to make quality improvement and cost containment decisions when dealing with prospective and capitated payments. Many consultants now say that the managed care plan with the best information system, not the best hospitals or physician groups, will win the largest share of any local health care market. Clinically based information on practice patterns and outcomes will allow physician groups to undertake extensive quality improvement activities that will produce better outcomes, document their ability to achieve them (and thus win contracts), and save costs by eliminating unnecessary care and expensive complications.

Unfortunately, most current clinical information is derived from claims data, which are often inaccurate and usually do not contain the type of clinical information required to engage in quality improvement activities. Thus, most advanced managed care organizations are making vast investments, on the order of tens of millions of dollars, in information systems. There is no single perfect system. The transition to an electronic medical record that contains all information on all patients does not yet exist. But no plan can afford to wait for such a mature system as the competition sweeps by them. Progressive investment is commencing today so that plans will know what to look for in systems of the future and can create what useful information is possible from claims data currently available.

## Systems

Care cannot be managed for lower cost and higher quality outcomes without some type of coordination of all of the above concepts. The dissipation of risk via large pools of patients, the collection and analysis of data, the provision of care under capitation, and the alignment of risk between providers cannot be undertaken by a small group of providers. Such activities must be organized into some type of coordinated system that can contract with an employer who does not have the expertise to provide such coordination.

Systems can be fully integrated into a single entity to include providers, inpatient institutions, and financing mechanisms. They can also be organized by contractual relationships. The key to the success for both situations is to be sure that incentives between the components are aligned in the same direction. If not, the components could be working at cross purposes, such as the hospital trying to keep beds full, while the insurer or health plan is trying to keep them empty so as not to spend prepaid dollars.

Alignment of incentives is critical, because that is where savings will be achieved. Again, this alignment and the savings it can produce can only be attained by an organized system, the health plan. If a provider group or institution is not a member of a health plan, it will not get access to patients. The only way for patients to fully choose where they will obtain care is to either have access to indemnity insurance, which because of its soaring cost is rapidly disappearing, or be eligible for Medicaid or Medicare. But even these government programs are being rapidly organized into risk-bearing managed care health plans that will direct patients to health plan providers and institutions.

### Competition

Even though the Clinton administration's version of health care reform, managed competition, died at the end of 1994, market reform is rapidly sweeping the nation. As care is organized into systems to reduce costs, these systems have progressively competed with each other to obtain patients. The fundamental and most measurable feature of this competition is cost; and the more organized and coordinated the system is, the more likely the cost can be successfully lowered.

Because this organized, market-based competition is succeeding in containing, and on the West Coast even lowering, the cost of care, legislated health care reform no longer matters. The only legislation so far produced has been minor insurance reform, and little more is anticipated in the near term. Market-driven competition organized through managed care will continue to be the mechanism of producing value for the purchaser. It is no longer sufficient to understand the concept of managed care as the intrusion of some third party into the decision making of a provider. Rather, managed care is the entrance of American medicine into the traditional American free enterprise system, a system that is based on competition.

### Value

Producing value is what managed care is all about. Value is the measured quality of the outcome, and of the service with which it is delivered, divided by the cost required to produce it. This is what competitive market systems are structured to produce: maximum quality and service at a minimum cost. While the focus of value is currently on cost, it will progressively move to documented quality and superior customer service. Systems and health plans that can produce value for employers and government programs will get the patients. Physicians and health care institutions that cannot provide comparatively lower cost, documentable (not presumed) quality, and excellent service will not get the patients, and will thus likely go out of business.

Business failure is the apparent fate of most academic medical centers and faculty practice plans. Why this is so and what can be done about it will be discussed next.

## The Impact of Managed Care on Faculty Practice Plans

Perhaps the most enduring feature of managed care is that it will generate constant and continuous change: Change is! The evolution to a health care delivery system that produces real value for purchasers will be increasingly rapid, profound, displacing, and extremely difficult for most academic faculties to endure. It entails a value base fundamentally different from that with which most faculty members have become ingrained. This clash of values not only will lead to entrenched resistance, but also will make it difficult for most faculty members to even understand what is occurring around them and why.

### Centralization

The inability to deal with change will make it extremely difficult for most faculty practice plans to institute the profound transformations required to withstand the aggressive competition being implemented by insurers, hospitals, and their town colleagues. The only way to rapidly and effectively overcome this resistance is to create effective and authoritative centralization.

One of the values of academic physicians that has traditionally served them well is autonomy. This concept is often translated into decentralized practice plans, or centralized plans where democracy or individual department veto can forestall a necessary market or contractual response. Faculty members' distrust of change and of each other inhibits the centralized authoritative decision making that the managed care marketplace demands. Most emerging health plans do not have the time and resources needed to draft and execute contracts for each specialty service, especially when they can easily be forged with competing multispecialty groups. Further, specialty services do not ordinarily have the expertise to negotiate with experienced health plan contract specialists.

To be competitive and attractive, a medical school's practice plans must be organized into a centralized governance that has the requisite expertise and independent authority to negotiate contracts and rates, as well as to undertake proactive programs and planning to make the practice plan an attractive partner.

Another reason for "corporate" or authoritative centralization is to pool resources and the decision making to utilize them. The plan needs to be able to hire knowledgeable expertise to position itself in the marketplace, as well as to be able to negotiate with health plans and HMOs. This type of human resource is rare, and thus expensive. Economy will be achieved, however, by utilizing this central expertise for all departments.

The plan has to make other expensive investments to make it attractive to health plans and patients. In particular, a primary care base will have to be acquired that can channel patients to specialists. Development of meaningful data to feed back to clinicians will also need to be financed. Planning and marketing are a basic requirement. Finally, capital will need to be expended on the development of new legal entities, and perhaps even a home-grown HMO, to effectively compete in the rapidly changing marketplace.

All of this requires a strong, centralized corporate authority that can "tax" department revenues for development purposes and that can appropriately divide up capitated prepayments. Further, the authority must be able to make decisions and develop plans unencumbered by the typical political dominance of various departments. The absence of such central authority means paralysis and parochial development, which in turn mean inability to compete.

## Primary Care Base

Probably the most fundamental flaw of most faculty practice plans is the lack of a dedicated primary care base. Specialists, who dominate faculty practice plans, will not have access to patients unless there is a primary care entry point. The magnitude of this need is being illustrated by highly advanced and integrated commercial health plans that are moving rapidly toward a 60 to 65 percent base of primary care physicians.

Strategies to obtain this base include purchasing private primary care practices, but this approach is expensive, requiring a substantial current capital reserve. Also, the practices for sale are not usually ones with the highest quality, which could prove very costly in the long run. Another strategy is to grow a primary care base within the academic faculty. This is a potentially powerful strategy, as the practice plan can often retain the best and the brightest from the generalist residencies. But this approach also requires substantial capital to competitively compensate such individuals and to purchase clinics in which to place them.

A final approach is to build outstanding referral relationships with private practice generalists and to develop contractual access to them. This is certainly the most economic approach, but such relationships are usually well in place with town specialists and contractual access may be extremely difficult. More likely, a combination of all three approaches will have to be pursued and will entail substantial capital outlay.

## Financial Partnership
Currently, in most faculty/hospital arrangements, it is the hospital that is the dominant financial resource. This, in turn, leads to difficult political relationships often dominated by conflict and lack of trust. But it is a rare faculty practice plan that has the capital needed to make the investments noted above. To succeed, the faculty practice plan must have as a financial partner either a hospital or a health plan insurer. Most state governments and research agencies are unable or unwilling to be a source of entrepreneurial investment for patient care.

While many faculty members would consider a partnership with an insurer or a commercial health plan to be a perversion of the academic mission, such a partnership is definitely worth considering. If the appropriate contractual safeguards can be included, such investments could rapidly move the faculty practice to the competitive forefront. Funding would be available to develop primary care; a source of good claims data would be available with which to document and improve clinical outcomes; and a foundation for referrals from outside the medical center could be enhanced. But, at some point, the investment will need a return, and the faculty plan will have to be accountable for this.

Much of the capital problem could be solved if the hospital and faculty practice plan budgets were integrated or at least highly coordinated. Potential for this usually exists through academic medical center governance. But, all too often, political considerations intervene, and market opportunity is lost while political infighting takes time and toll to work out. If this structural problem can be solved up front, either through a central decision maker or through development of an effective physician-hospital organization with shared governance, swift action and the financing for it can be achieved. This is probably preferable to an outside financial backer, as inherent values are more compatible and the room for financial mistakes is much larger.

## Enhancing Cost Effectiveness
The shift to capitation, especially for full risk prepayment, is as profound a change for faculty practice plans as is the shift to primary care. As noted previously, most plans, centralized or not, evolve around productivity and the piecework revenue it produces. This stimulates clinicians, particularly proceduralists, to provide all the services that are even marginally appropriate for patients. Under capitated prepayment, a medical group will enhance retained revenue by undertaking only services that are clearly indicated and appropriate. Thus, doing less and keeping required services at the least expensive level will produce more income. To encourage this type of behavior, individuals can no longer be paid for what they do. Rather they need to be compensated for covering the risk of all potential appropriate care in their areas of medical responsibility. The processes for determining what payments should

be made to each area, ensuring that the distribution is actuarially fair, and appropriately rewarding primary care is fraught with conflict and resentment. Again, only strong, creditable, and authoritative central leadership can provide this.

Learning to operate appropriately within such financial constraints is another gigantic leap. This requires collection and interpretation of cost data and willingness to have such data on practice patterns documented. Length of stay, urgent care visits, number of procedures, etc. must all be periodically collected, analyzed, and fed back to the clinicians who control them. This, in turn, requires faculty members to use the information to examine their practice patterns and to find areas in which practices can be improved. While this occurs as a rule with residents, most faculty members are loathe to have their care monitored.

### Report Cards on Quality and Service
While cost remains the focus of most health care reform activities, it is clear that employers are concerned that their employees continue to receive excellent care and service. Because they readily recognize that they do not have the expertise to ensure this themselves, they are turning to consultants and new national organizations, such as the National Committee on Quality Assurance and its Health Employer Data and Information Set (HEDIS). These entities are developing "report cards" that ascertain patient satisfaction, standard processes of care, and some basic outcomes of care. No longer will it suffice to produce low-cost care, especially as price begins to level out in the future. Rather, each provider group and allied health plan will have to document quality of care and excellence of service. Outcomes on these measures will then be used to qualify for bids from employers, as well as for selection of plans by patients.

It will thus be incumbent on faculty practice plans to collect all relevant data and measures. They will also have to ensure that patients have easy, timely, and friendly access to faculty physicians, being sure that resident care is only an option for the patient to choose, not a standard. Again, collecting and demonstrating data will require investment, as will staffing access to ambulatory care that can measure up to the levels of service that are second nature to competing private practices.

Finally, faculty members will have to develop a sense of "customer" service and accountability that they have traditionally been able to escape. Clinics can no longer be canceled at the convenience of the faculty member, and routinely placing a fellow or resident between the full professor and the patient will drive away health plan enrollees. Establishing such standards and enforcing them will require a strong centralized authority that can overcome the protests of even the chair of surgery.

### Timing
Because faculty practice plans are more a political pantheon than a corporate commission, the pace of change is usually guarded and very deliberate. There is also a "welfare" mentality that believes that, at the last moment, federal and state governments will unleash a deus ex machina and deliver the academic faculty from financial distress. Unfortunately the political climate is moving in the opposite direction, and many legislators believe that it was the medical schools that placed the nation in its current dilemma by training too many specialists. If a large number of schools fail, some relief might be forthcoming. But, in the meantime, facul-

ty practice plans and academic medical centers must fend for themselves and do so rapidly. While the most radical competition is occurring on the West coast, many East coast cities are leapfrogging the intermediate stages of managed care and are evolving highly competitive managed care plans that are dominating their marketplaces.

Moving rapidly to centralize, to create access to capital, and to develop a solid primary care base is exceedingly difficult under the best of circumstances for any health care providing organization. But "rapid" and "aggressive" must be watch words, or a revenue-producing patient base will be lost.

## The Future

While it is apparent that faculty practice plans, as currently structured, will not do well in a managed care environment, there is reason for optimism. First, even though they may be loosely organized, most faculty practice plans are part of multispecialty groups. This will actually assist the process of forging closer links between departments. Also, most plans are highly integrated, at least in form and geography, with academic hospitals. This integration and their shared mission will assist plans and hospitals in working through such issues as capitation distribution and incentive alignment for cost control .

Second, even though most practice plans have minimal primary care membership, medical schools are the training places of primary care physicians. As primary care physicians become progressively more rare and in demand, medical schools should be able to hold on to the best and the brightest. as long as they can pay them on a market basis.

Third, many academic hospitals are a source of funds for primary care expansion and information systems development. The only problem is in creating genuine access to those funds. But as academic hospitals become increasingly imperiled by the competition, sharing reserves should become significantly easier.

Fourth, once faculty practice plans learn to collect health services data and manipulate them into information, the research experience should greatly assist faculty practice plans in studying and documenting improved patient outcomes. In time, this will be of significant advantage in the local marketplace.

The transition to managed care will be difficult and painful. Health care is undergoing much of the same transitional difficulties that airlines did when they became deregulated. Many hospitals and providers will go out of business. But providers that can organize highly competitive systems that produce efficiency and enhance quality and service, the goals of managed care, will thrive. Faculty practice plans that can face up to the difficult transition process by providing strong and centralized leadership, respecting and financing primary care and acquiring and acting on practice pattern data, will be the plans that survive and ensure survival of the traditional missions and values of academic medicine.

*Martin E. Hickey, MD, MS, FACPE, is Chief Medical Officer, Lovelace Health Systems, and Adjunct Associate Professor of Medicine, University of New Mexico, Albuquerque.*

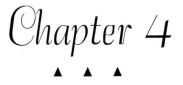

# Chapter 4

▲  ▲  ▲

## Teaching in the Faculty Practice Setting

by Mark Kushner, MD, Shari L. Bornstein, MD, MPH,
and Roger Hand, MD

*M*edical school clinical training began in this country with the apprenticeship system. "Faculty practices" were the predominant, if not the only, training sites. The growth of medical schools and, ultimately, of hospitals as places where acute care was rendered shifted the site of clinical education from patient homes or practitioner offices to the medical science "laboratory" or modern hospital. The inpatient clinical clerkship reached its zenith at the beginning of the 20th Century under Osler at Johns Hopkins. It has continued to be the usual form of undergraduate clinical education.

Over the past several decades, for economic reasons and because of technical advancement in medical care, there has been a shift from in-hospital care to ambulatory care. Inpatient stays are shorter, and patients' conditions are more complex. This makes the student clerkship experience less satisfying.[1,2] Societal health care needs are now better accomplished by fostering ambulatory primary care. This was recognized early on by Flexner and more recently by the Association of American Medical Colleges in the report of its Panel on the General Professional Education of the Physician and College Preparation for Medicine (GPEP).[2]

Surveys of medical school and residency graduates have shown that graduates perceive they had inadequate preparation for primary care and ambulatory care roles because of deficient curricula and clinical exposure.[3-5] Since the GPEP report's publication, most medical schools have increased training in ambulatory care for students and residents. With the increase has come the realization that teaching in the outpatient setting is quite different from teaching in the inpatient setting. While the three basic functions of a clinical faculty—modeling, supervision, and consultation[6]—are the same in both settings, the teaching behaviors used to accomplish these functions differ.[7,8] The most obvious change is the size of the learning group. In the classic inpatient teaching encounter, a faculty member teaches several learners at once, typically a senior resident, one or more junior residents, and several students. In an outpatient teaching encounter, there is usually only one learner in the group, be it a resident or student.

This one-on-one situation has forced medical schools to increase the number of sites for teaching ambulatory care. Twenty years ago, a typical department of medicine might have had a single resident-driven general medicine clinic to provide ambulatory care experience for its trainees. Now, that same department will have multiple sites on and off campus for both students and residents. Faculty practice sites, whether for primary care or specialty care, are convenient and necessary for instruction.

Most faculty practices were set up to be just that—sites where faculty members could see their own patients, unencumbered by students and residents. These teaching sites have experienced problems: lack of space, poor patient mix, poor patient acceptance, loss of faculty time for other academic activities, and lost revenues. Most of these problems are also found in private practices that have been recruited as teaching sites. While faculty practices may differ markedly from private academic practices in many management aspects, they probably are similar insofar as problems related to teaching are concerned.

**Lack of Space.** A medical student requires a dedicated examination room for the time he or she is in clinic.[9] Residents ideally would use more than one examination room but may spend only 25 percent of their time in examination rooms in patient contact.[10] Third-year students may see as few as one or two patients per session,[11] while fourth-year students may see three or four.[12] Estimates of resident productivity indicate they produce only 40-54 percent of what a faculty member produced.[13] In subspecialty clinics, being seen by the resident physician rather than by the attending increases the length of the patients' visit by 18 minutes, or 25 percent.[14] Few faculty practice sites have sufficient examination rooms to accommodate students and residents easily when the rooms are used for so few patients.

**Poor Patient Mix.** Primary care faculty practices, especially those on the main campuses of large university medical centers, may have a limited patient mix. Hand *et al.*[15] showed that only 8 of the leading 25 diagnoses on the National Ambulatory Care Health Survey were reasonably represented in primary care clinics at a large university center. Common diagnoses, such as low back pain, ischemic heart disease, and sinusitis, are often cared for in specialty clinics. In addition, urgent care conditions, such as urinary tract infections and lacerations, may be seen in emergency departments rather than in faculty practices, especially in academic medical centers in urban areas.

**Poor Patient Acceptance.** At a faculty practice site, patients may expect services to be provided by their regular attending physician. Being seen by a student or resident may not always be acceptable to them. The problems faced by patients in the teaching site may include anger from the delay caused by teaching and confusion as to who is responsible for their care.[8] A survey of academic private practice sites found that most patient refusals were related to the nature of the medical problem, e.g., psychiatric or sexual. The survey reports that most patients enjoyed the extra attention and liked taking part in the students' education.[16] A careful introduction of the student to the patient by the attending physician will usually avoid problems.[12]

**Loss of Faculty Time for Other Academic Activities.** Teaching ambulatory care requires time, a commodity in short supply for many academic physicians. The presence of a student in internal medicine or family practice offices adds one hour or 20-25 percent to a teacher's clinic session.[16] This holds true for other specialties represented in traditional third-year clerkships.[17] Rabinowitz[18] comments how faculty members who support these programs have little time for research and have difficulty with promotion. In his program (at Jefferson Medical College, one of the oldest ambulatory care clerkships), most faculty members are successful in being promoted in a clinical track. There are other reports of no loss of time or productivity by faculty members.[19-20] In one study, investigators found that most preceptors reported an increased amount of time at work with no loss of income.[21]

**Loss of Revenues.** Early studies on teaching ambulatory care showed that faculty teaching practices, while inefficient, were marginally profitable because of the lower costs of student and resident providers.[22,23] Garg *et al.*[24] estimated that teaching up to two students each year cost practice sites more than $20,000/year in lost revenues. Recent estimates of costs per student per half-day session are $77[17] and $50 to $100.[12] This is not substantially different from cost estimates taken from the late 1970s.[23] Costs for residents are less, but their productivity is still well below that of attending physicians.[15] However, some recent studies also suggest that residents, especially more senior ones, may be nearly as productive as faculty members in terms of patients seen and duration of visits.[25]

In facing these and lesser problems, clerkship directors and residency program directors have made recommendations for teaching in the faculty practice setting, among them that preceptors devote their assigned time entirely to teaching, rather than trying to mix supervision with direct care to their own patients.[10,26] Other factors important to success include enthusiasm for the program on the part of institutional leadership and a structured curriculum.[18] Appropriate evaluation is especially important for both student[27-29] and resident[30,31] programs.

## Model Programs

Several recent publications have dealt with these issues in detail and with innovative solutions or hard outcome measures related to finances and evaluation: An internal medicine residency training program based at an HMO at Harvard Medical School,[32] an internal medicine residency training program at the University of Illinois Champaign-Urbana College of Medicine,[13] a third-year student program at the University of Oregon,[33] and a longitudinal primary care program at the University of Illinois at Chicago.

**Dealing with Poor Patient Mix: Structuring Residents' Panels.** The Harvard Community Health Plan (now the Pilgrim-Harvard Community Health Plan) recognized that selection of a panel of patients for a resident may be random or may be influenced by factors other than the teaching value of a patient's case.[32] It devised a curriculum-based patient assignment system. Fifteen diagnostic or management conditions in internal medicine were selected. Attending physicians preferentially assigned patients with these conditions from their own panels to residents. Extra effort was placed on getting patients' acceptance of assignments. The attending physician reassumed care of patient in the absence of the resident, for instances during a resident's assignment to intensive care or emergency medicine. The advantages of this plan are:

▲ Residents begin their ambulatory care rotation with a panel containing significant "pathology."

▲ Preceptors can take better advantage of teaching encounters because they have some prior knowledge of patients.

▲ Preceptors and residents are focused on a defined curriculum of common conditions throughout the rotation.

**Lost Revenues: Paying the Preceptor.** The Carle Clinic at the University of Illinois Champaign-Urbana College of Medicine "taxes" attending physician revenues (from patients for whom the attending physicians provide supervision for resident services, for example, when their patients are hospitalized on the teaching service) to set up a residency account to pay attendings for teaching ambulatory care.[13] Preceptors are paid at about the same rate they would receive if they were seeing their own patients in the absence of residents. Taking into account the lower productivity of residents, the clinic uses a ratio of one preceptor to three residents to ensure that patient service revenues to the practice are maintained.

**Lost Revenues: The Cost of a Single Student.** The University of Oregon assigns students to academic rural private practices. Investigators surveyed 22 teaching sites, each of which had one student, for gross charges, outpatient and inpatient charges, and total visits.[33] There was a drop in daily charges of $53 (with a standard deviation of $315) and a drop in total visits per day of 0.2 (with a standard deviation of 3.1). Neither drop was statistically significant. Overall, increased workload and lost revenues were real but small.

**A Structured Curriculum for Students.** At the University of Illinois at Chicago, we have established a structured curriculum for a three-year primary care clerkship. This was intended to replace a one-month block rotation during the fourth year. Analysis of the effects of these block rotation clerkships has shown variable results. Students valued the experience and said it increased their appreciation of primary care. There was, however, only modest improvement in the chance of the student choosing a career in primary care, because many students had already made plans for residency training.[11,29]

The faculty abandoned the block rotation and moved toward a longitudinal primary care clerkship. In 1991, after three years of planning, the curriculum committee established the program for years one through three of the medical school curriculum. The program was piloted for three years, with increasing numbers of volunteer students, and then made a mandatory part of the curriculum, with full student participation for the class entering in 1994.

The main goal of the program is to introduce medical students early in their training to primary care medicine as practiced in the ambulatory setting. This is accomplished by assigning students to primary care practitioners (general internists, family practitioners, and pediatricians) in a one-to-one ratio. Although a variety of practice sites are used (university clinics, neighborhood clinics, and private offices), nearly all full-time primary care providers involved in faculty practices were assigned one or more students. The longitudinal aspect of the program was seen as crucial in giving students an experience in continuous care of a

**Table 1.** Educational Themes of a Primary Care Clerkship

▲ Continuity of care of patients and families

▲ Observational and perceptual skills

▲ Interviewing skills

▲ Importance of cultural factors in patient care

▲ Problem-solving as a developmental process

▲ Importance of nonphysician health care providers

▲ Importance of the community in health care

panel of patients. Specific educational themes run through all three years of the program (table 1, above). The student-patient encounter is the teaching opportunity, and students assume greater care responsibilities as their ability and progress merit them.

A curriculum was developed for each of the program's three years. The topics, in the order they are introduced to the students, are listed in table 2, page 28. Because of the diversity of the faculty members involved, curriculum implementation sessions are held to familiarize them with the program. The curriculum is designed to be more a guide than a specific list of required activities. However, it does contain specific readings, suggested student activities, and suggested teaching points for each topic. The basic unit of instruction is a one-on-one session with student and preceptor at the primary care site. Exposure to all aspects of the physician's practice—including time with nonphysician health care providers—is encouraged. In the first year, the student attends one session per month; in the second year, attendance is every two weeks; in the third year, the student attends weekly.

The program has expanded from 51 students in the first pilot year of 1991 to more than 300 students and 250 preceptors four years later. It is now a required clerkship, and, in two years, it will involve all students in medical school years one to three. The course has required a considerable amount of faculty time. Organizational, recruitment, and monitoring activities are done by the Department of Medical Education. Faculty development has been a major effort. Activities include a monthly newsletter and CME sessions covering curriculum implementation, feedback to students, and teaching skills.

The preceptors and students are surveyed annually. Preceptors enjoy the experience of role-modeling and believe they are contributing to students' professional development and influencing them to choose primary care careers. The students are not seen as significant time or cost drains to practices, whether faculty practices, true private practices, or community clinics.

**Table 2.** Specific Topics for Each Year
in a Longitudinal Primary Care Clerkship

**First Year Curriculum**
- ▲ Basic interviewing skills
- ▲ Doctor-patient relationship
- ▲ Illness versus disease
- ▲ Patient's experience of illness
- ▲ Impact of patient's and doctor's culture and ethnicity
- ▲ Doctor's role as a primary care provider
- ▲ Role of the community in the patient's care
- ▲ Role of family in the patient's care

**Second Year Curriculum**
- ▲ Intermediate interviewing skills
- ▲ Health risk factors and health promotion behaviors
- ▲ Continuity of care
- ▲ Developmental stages and natural history of chronic ambulatory disease
- ▲ Influence of cultural background on health (review)
- ▲ Understanding health problems of a community (review)
- ▲ Primary care in the community: working with other providers (review)

**Third Year Curriculum**
- ▲ Advanced interviewing skills
- ▲ Continuity of care (review)
- ▲ Clinical exposure, observational skills, problem solving
- ▲ Primary care physician as member of patient care team (review)
- ▲ Wellness, health promotion, and disease prevention

The preceptors expressed a need for help from the Department of Medical Education with teaching techniques, feedback and evaluation, and handling personality-related student problems.

Student satisfaction is high, especially regarding the mentor relationships established. They believe the clerkship enhance their academic and clinical performance overall. In particular, they see an improvement in relating to patients, in overcoming nervousness, and in listening and interviewing skills. Students see one to three patients each session and spend the majority of the session with their preceptor. The curriculum is felt to be helpful but difficult to adapt to the patients seen in the office. Despite provision of detailed written guidelines for the curriculum, with references, some preceptors did not adhere to them. This is regarded as a drawback by students.

One of our faculty practice sites involved in the longitudinal care clerkship is Internal Medicine Faculty Associates. It is located on the medical school campus. It is a busy practice with more than 14,000 visits per year. More than 90 percent of the patients are insured, with a growing percentage of managed cared patients. Faculty members act as preceptors for students on a regular basis at this site. Most patient contacts are regularly scheduled appointments. However, because it is a comprehensive managed care practice on the campus, students can work with preceptors on all aspects of the practice. Potentially, a student has the opportunity to see the full spectrum of a general internist's practice: hospital rounds, emergency department visits, calls back to patient, and office visits. With regular and frequent visits to the clinic, the student has the opportunity to follow the patient longitudinally and to appreciate the evolution of disease and the doctor-patient relationship. In this program, students have their first patient encounter; this is their first opportunity to wear a white coat, use a stethoscope, and take a blood pressure.

Other benefits to the student include participating for an extended period with one preceptor—receiving one-on-one attention. There is immediate feedback on histories, physical findings, oral and written presentations, and clinical decision making. In an academic setting, the students can see how attending physicians interact with other students, residents, and fellows, which can demystify these relationships for students in the preclinical years and allow them to understand better what will be expected of them in the future.

The difficulties that such long-term programs pose for students are primarily related to scheduling conflicts and choice of preceptors. While all clerkship directors are required to release students in their third year rotations for weekly ambulatory care clinics, students sometimes feel a conflict with ward responsibilities. For example, it can be difficult for students to get away during a busy surgery rotation. The second problem is that, while faculty preceptors for the Longitudinal Care Program are selected because of their interest in or talent for teaching, a particular student and preceptor may not be compatible. Given the nature of the one-on-one relationship, this usually requires a change of preceptor.

There are pros and cons for the faculty preceptor as well. Most university-based faculty members enjoy teaching and have spent at least part of their careers in teaching. The Longitudinal Primary Care program gives faculty members an opportunity to model the art of medicine along the lines of the old apprenticeship. While these benefits are personally rewarding for preceptors, they have been perceived as time-consuming and labor-intensive. In the managed care setting with prepaid capitation, revenues are more easily maintained, but the preceptors invariably spend more time in the clinic on a teaching day. To minimize this, for purposes of maintaining staff as well as of physician satisfaction, we decrease a preceptor's patient load on a teaching day. We also limit teaching sessions to one or two half-days week. A flexible and responsive scheduling system allows us to compensate for lost visits on teaching days with slightly increased bookings on nonteaching days. This minimizes the impact of teaching on patient care services. With a capitated patient base, there is no impact on revenues.

## Conclusions

Experience indicates that most of the difficulties of teaching in faculty practices can be overcome. They certainly can be dealt with in academic private practices, where having a student for the full academic year or for a limited part of the year is accepted by faculty preceptors. Lost revenues can be minimized. Rewards for excellence in teaching, such as promotion and tenure, should be achievable as more and more medical schools recognize the importance of instruction in ambulatory medicine. Other barriers, such as lack of space and poor patient mix, can be overcome with appropriate practice management. Finally, structured curricula, delivered by skilled faculty members in practice settings attuned to the needs of students and residents, can enhance the value of the clerkship. Longitudinal care experiences, whether in faculty practice sites or in other academic practice settings, should help prepare the next generation of physicians for their roles in providing high-quality ambulatory and primary care.

## References

1. Schroeder SA. Expanding the site of clinical education: Moving beyond the hospital walls. *Journal of General Internal Medicine* 3 (2 suppl):S5-14, March-April 1988.

2. *Physicians for the Twenty-First Century: The GPEP Report. Report of the Panel on the General Professional Education of the Physician and College Preparation for Medicine.* Washington, D.C.: Association of American Medical Colleges, 1984.

3. Gary, N. "Barriers to Medical Education in the Ambulatory Setting." *Journal of Medical Education* 62(6):527-9, June 1987.

4. Linn, L., and others. "Evaluation of Ambulatory Care Training by Graduates of Internal Medicine Residencies." *Journal of Medical Education* 61(4):293-302, April 1986.

5. Mandel, J., and others. "Preparation for Practice in Internal Medicine: A Study of Ten Years of Residency Graduates." *Archives of Internal Medicine* 148(4):853-6, April 1988.

6. Biddle, B., and others. "A Promising Approach to Teaching Primary Care in the Ambulatory Setting." *Academic Medicine* 67(7):457, July 1992.

7. Loftus, T., and others. "Faculty Perceptions of Effective Ambulatory Care Teaching." *Journal of General Internal Medicine* 8(10):575-7, Oct. 1993.

8. Lesky, L., and Borkan, S. "Strategies to Improve Teaching in the Ambulatory Medicine Setting." *Archives of Internal Medicine* 150(10):2133-7, Oct. 1990.

9. Brzezinski, W. "An Ambulatory Care Internal Medicine Rotation for Third-Year Medical Students." *Academic Medicine* 65(11):717, Nov. 1990.

10. Lawrence, S., and others. "Students' Time Allocation in a Required Third-Year Ambulatory Care Clerkship." *Academic Medicine* 69(1):60-1, Jan. 1994.

11. Papadakis, M., and Kagawa, M. "A Randomized, Controlled Pilot Study of Placing Third-Year Medical Clerks in a Continuity Clinic." *Academic Medicine* 68(11):845-7, Nov. 1993.

12. Shore, W., and Rodnick, J. "A Required Fourth-Year Ambulatory Clerkship: A 10-Year Experience with Family Practice and Primary Care Internal Medicine Sites." *Family Medicine* 25(1):34-40, Jan. 1993.

13. Kirby, R. "Financing Residency Education in the Ambulatory Setting: A Private Practice Model." *Journal of General Internal Medicine* 6(6):579-82, Nov.-Dec. 1991.

14. Gamble, J., and Lee, R. "Investigating Whether Education of Residents in a Group Practice Increases the Length of the Outpatient Visit." *Academic Medicine* 66(8):492-3, Aug. 1991.

15. Hand, R., and others. "Patient Mix in the Primary Ambulatory Care Clinics of an Academic Medical Center." *Academic Medicine* 68(10):803-5, Oct. 1993.

16. Packman, C., and others. "The Rochester Practice-Based Experience. An Experiment in Medical Education." *Archives of Internal Medicine* 154(11):1253-60, June 1994.

17. Vanek, E., and others. "Assessing the Resources Needed to Provide Ambulatory Care Experiences to Medical Students." *Academic Medicine* 68(3):202-3, March 1993.

18. Rabinowitz, H. Sixteen Years' Experience with a Required Third-Year Family Medicine Clerkship at Jefferson Medical College." *Academic Medicine* 67(3):150-6, March 1992.

19. Hansen, L., and Talley, R. "South Dakota's Third-Year Program of Integrated Clerkships in Ambulatory Care Settings." *Academic Medicine* 67(12):817-9, Dec. 1992.

20. Kearl, G., and Mainous, A. "Physicians' Productivity and Teaching Responsibilities." *Academic Medicine* 68(2):166-7, Feb. 1993.

21. Vinson, D., and Paden, C. "The Effect of Teaching Medical Students on Private Practitioners' Workloads." *Academic Medicine* 69(3):237-8, March 1994.

22. Kosecoff, J., and others. "Providing Primary General Medical Care in University Hospitals: Efficiency and Cost." *Annals of Internal Medicine* 107(3):399-405, Sept. 1987.

23. Delbanco, T., and Calkins, D. "The Costs and Financing of Ambulatory Medical Education." *Journal of General Internal Medicine* 3(2 suppl):S34-43, March-April 1988.

24. Garg, M., and others. "Primary Care Teaching Physicians' Losses of Productivity and Revenue at Three Ambulatory Care Centers." *Academic Medicine* 66(6):348-53, June 1991.

25. Gilchrist, V., and others. "Does Family Practice at Residency Teaching Sites Reflect Community Practice?" *Journal of Family Practice* 37(6):555-63, Dec. 1993.

26. Dauphinee, W. "Clinical Education: The legacy of Osler Revisited." *Academic Medicine* 65(9 suppl):S68-73, Sept. 1990 .

27. Harris, L., and others. "Development and Evaluation of a Required Ambulatory Medicine Clerkship." *Academic Medicine* 66(9):511-2, Sept. 1991.

28. Grum, C., and Woolliscroft, J. "What Are Students Learning during Ambulatory Rotations? Implications for Generalist Education." *Academic Medicine* 69(5):420, May 1994.

29. Rucker, L., and others. "Impact of Ambulatory Care Clerkship on the Attitudes of Students from Five Classes (1985-1989) toward Primary Care." *Academic Medicine* 66(10):620-2, Oct. 1991.

30. Moran, M., and Nanda, J. "Primary Care Residency Programme Evaluation: An Analysis of Three Resident Cohorts." *Medical Teacher* 14(2):223-9, Spring 1992.

31. Blankfield, R., and others. "Continuity of Care in a Family Practice Residency Program. Impact on Physician Satisfaction." *Journal of Family Practice* 31(1):69-73, July 1990.

32. Kirby, A., and Bush, G. "Assigning Patients According to Curriculum: A Strategy for Improving Ambulatory Care Residency Training." *Academic Medicine* 69(9):717-9, Sept. 1994.

33. Fields, S., and others. "Impact of the Presence of a Third-Year Medical Student on Gross Charges and Patient Volumes in 22 Rural Community Practices." *Academic Medicine* 69(10 suppl):S87-9, Oct. 1994.

*Mark Kushner, MD, Shari L. Bornstein, MD, and Roger Hand, MD, are Assistant Professor, Instructor, and Professor, respectively, Department of Medicine, College of Medicine, University of Illinois at Chicago.*

# Chapter 5

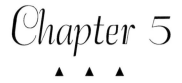

## Faculty Practice Plan
## Governance and Management

### by William H. Frishman, MD

Clinical departments in medical schools are complex organizations that employ hundreds of full-time faculty members and are responsible for large educational, clinical, and research enterprises. These departments have come under increasing strain from changing patterns of practice and financial compensation, and decreased funding for research.

In recent years, state and local government appropriations for medical school departments have decreased, as have parent university support, endowments, and teaching and training grants. However, practice plan revenues have exhibited strong growth and now account for one-third of medical school revenues. This reflects a 10 percent increase over 1992-1993 earnings in current dollars, and a 6.8 percent increase in inflation-adjusted dollars.[1]

Of the dollars that are generated for medical services rendered by faculty, two-thirds are generated by practice plans.[1] How these revenues are handled to support academic programs and faculty salaries varies from institution to institution.

In this chapter, I will discuss the practice plan developed for full-time practicing faculty in the Department of Medicine at the Albert Einstein College of Medicine and at Montefiore Medical Center. Faculty members receive their base pay from either the medical school or the hospital. However, all practicing faculty belong to a single practice plan, which is described below. Other specialties have their own practice plans, which are similar generically to the Department of Medicine plan but differ in the particulars.

Montefiore Medical Center (MMC) and the Albert Einstein College of Medicine (AECOM) have entered into an agreement providing that AECOM employees in the Department of Medicine and MMC employees in the Department of Medicine practice under a faculty practice plan operated by Montefiore. The agreement provides terms and conditions applicable to the plan, including definitions of, among other things, "covered practitioners" and "covered practice activities."

# Income

The agreement between MMC and AECOM provides, among other things, that all practice income derived from any patient care activities (including income for interpretation of tests), either on or off campus, must be billed and collected through the plan. Any practice income paid directly to a physician must be turned over to the plan immediately. Any payments related to outside speaking engagements and work for the National Institutes of Health and other not-for-profit organizations must be accounted for in accord with the rules and regulations of Yeshiva University, the parent organization for AECOM, for its faculty and with those of MMC for its employees.

The amount of the practitioner's base salary supported from plan funds and any supplemental distributions from the plan are paid to the practitioner by his or her employer (MMC or AECOM) from plan funds. In the case of practitioners employed by AECOM, MMC remits to AECOM plan funds comprising any base salary support from practice revenues together with related fringe benefit costs. MMC also remits to AECOM plan funds comprising any supplemental distributions of plan earnings owed to practitioners employed by AECOM. For some AECOM employees, plan funds remitted to AECOM for supplements will include, in addition to the supplement amount to be distributed to each such AECOM employee, an amount to cover all fringe benefit costs related to the supplement (the additional amount being paid from the department component of plan collections). An exception is the tax-deferred annuity contribution component of plan collections, which is charged against and paid from the supplement amount due to the AECOM employee. For AECOM practitioners in the latter group who do not accept an offer of employment by MMC, all fringe benefit costs relating to supplemental distributions are charged against and paid from the individual's supplemental distribution amount remitted to AECOM. No additional plan funds are remitted to AECOM for this purpose.

# Overhead

Overhead is paid to MMC from the department's component of plan income. In the base year of the plan, which runs July 1 through June 30, overhead was 6.5 percent of gross practice income. In each subsequent year, the overhead charge is calculated by adjusting the dollar amount of overhead that was charged in the base year by an inflation factor determined by the Montefiore Medical Center Office of Professional Services for application to all faculty practice plans. Rent for Department of Medicine practice space at AECOM is paid by MMC from the overhead it collects from the plan. Any additional rent is charged directly to the department.

# President's Fund

A charge of 15.5 percent of all nonprocedural income is made for the benefit of the MMC President's Fund. Procedural income is income for such services as cardiac catheter-izations, pulmonary function tests, and the like. Procedural income in the gastrointestinal division and all income, except capitation, generated by renal division physicians is considered to be nonprocedural. Services are classified as procedural and nonprocedural income in other divisions in accordance with the classifications for those divisions in effect on June 30 of the base year. Any changes in those classifications, and classification of any new services, is subject to MMC's oversight responsibility for management of the plan.

## Distribution Formula

### Procedural Income
All procedural income is retained by the Department of Medicine for support of its programs, in accordance with the conditions for departmental funds specified below. The chairman of the department of medicine may use procedural income for compensation in addition to base salary and in addition to supplemental distributions of nonprocedural income, with such arrangements being reviewed at the department's annual budget meeting. However, procedural income in the pulmonary division is used first to support base salaries and then, in instances approved by the chairman, for guaranteed supplements that are reviewed at the department's annual budget meeting.

### Nonprocedural Income
Of the gross collections of nonprocedural income generated by a practitioner, 60 percent is used to pay the practitioner a supplemental distribution, up to a maximum of 30 percent over the practitioner's base salary. As mentioned earlier, 15.5 percent of gross collections go to the President's Fund, and the balance of gross collections go to the Departmental Fund (see below).

After a practitioner has earned, as a supplement, 30 percent over his or her base salary, collections of nonprocedural income that he or she has generated are distributed as follows: 40 percent are used to pay the practitioner a supplemental distribution above the maximum of 30 percent, up to a maximum of 60 percent over the practitioner's base salary (inclusive of any fringe benefit costs); 15.5 percent goes to the President's Fund referred to above, and the balance goes to the Departmental Fund.

Supplemental distribution cannot be more than 60 percent over the pertinent practitioner's base salary, unless approved in writing by the department chairman. After a practitioner has earned supplements of 60 percent over his or her base salary, additional collections of nonprocedural income that the practitioner generates may, at the discretion of the chairman, be distributed to pay the practitioner a supplemental distribution above the 60 percent maximum at a rate of 20 percent of such additional collections; 15.5 percent of such additional collections go to the President's Fund and the remainder go to the Department Fund.

In recruiting new practitioners for employment in the department, the chairman may require practitioners to earn a portion of their respective base salaries (including guarnateed supplement, if any) from practice activities and require that the portion be collected before any supplemental distribution (or any distribution of guaranteed supplements) are made. In such cases, 78 percent of the collections are applied to base salary (including guaranteed supplement, if any) plus related fringe benefits; 15.5 percent goes to the President's Fund, and 6.5 percent goes to the Departmental Fund, from which overhead is paid. Thereafter, distributions are made as described earlier in this section. Certain currently employed practitioners are required to earn and collect a portion of their base salaries (including guaranteed supplement, if any) before any supplemental distribution (or any distribution of guaranteed supplements) is made to the practitioner. In such cases, 80 percent of collections is applied to base salary (including guaranteed supplement, if any) plus related fringe benefits; 15.5 percent goes to the President's Fund, and 4.5 percent goes to the Departmental Fund. Changes in the requirement that any specific practitioner earn a proportion of his or her base salary is reviewed at the annual departmental budget meeting by the institution that is the employer of the practitioner in question.

Before the plan was implemented, there were certain previously agreed-upon distribution arrangements for specific practitioners that varied from the general arrangements then in effect at MMC and AECOM for the practitioners' respective Department of Medicine practice plans. Those arrangements were allowed to continue, even when there was a variance between existing arrangements and the new plan rules. Arrangements in effect on July 1st that are at variance from these rules ("variances") may be applied to newly hired practitioners whose employments and economic practice circumstances are, and to other practitioners whose employment and economic practice circumstances are or become, substantially similar to the employment and economic practice circumstances of those to whom the particular variance was applicable on June 30th.

### Departmental Funds
Departmental funds may be allocated by the chairman to support the programs of the Division of Medicine in which such funds were earned or to support other needs of the department as a whole. Their use is in accordance with policies and procedures in effect at MMC and AECOM prior to implementation of the plan, provided use is consistent with provisions of the plan agreement. As with other matters, the conditions for use of departmental funds must be presented annually for approval to the administration of the two institutions at departmental budget meetings.

## Conclusion
In an era in which funding for academic departments of medicine is being curtailed by decreased funding from extramural grant sources, physician practices have become an even more important part of financing. We have been able to combine under one umbrella the private practice efforts from internal medicine faculty working in a predominantly research educational setting (Albert Einstein College of Medicine) and those of clinical faculty working in the university hospital (Montefiore Hospital). The plan described here has provided increased funding for faculty salary, research and educational endeavors so that the major missions of the medical center (patient care, research, education) can be maintained and even augmented.

## Reference
1. Ganem, J., and others. "Review of Medical School Finances, 1993-1994." *JAMA* 274(9):723-30, Sept. 6, 1995.

*William H. Frishman, MD, is Professor and Associate Chairman, Department Of Medicine, Albert Einstein College Of Medicine/Montefiore Medical Center, New York, New York.*

# Chapter 6

▲  ▲  ▲

## The Faculty Practice Plan
## in a Public Teaching Hospital

by William L. Boddie, MD

## Background

*Faculty practice plans have been more traditional in academic medical centers than in public teaching hospitals.*

It has been widely accepted that faculty practice plans have been traditional to academic medical centers. Although not widespread, application in public teaching hospitals has also been documented. Published reports have revealed successful plans in Baltimore City Hospital[1] and in New York.[2] Plans have existed in several California public teaching hospitals (Modesto, Merced, Fresno, San Bernardino, and Bakersfield).

*The model presented in this chapter is the Family Practice Program in Modesto, CA, which is affiliated with the University of California-Davis.*

Stanislaus Medical Center, a 132-bed public hospital in Modesto, California, was established in 1892. It provides medical services to the county's indigent population. In 1975, the hospital received approval to establish a family practice residency training program. The following year, the residency affiliated with the University of California at Davis School of Medicine. From 1975 to 1982, the hospital contracted with full-time faculty for the provision of medical services to county patients and for teaching services to the residents.

*The faculty practice plan was developed to facilitate faculty retention and recruitment.*

Compensation of the hospital-based faculty was significantly lower than and not competitive with the income of community physicians, particularly procedure-oriented specialists. As a result, faculty members were being lured away from the hospital by the higher compensation of private practice. In addition, recruitment was becoming more difficult. The financially strapped county could not practically or politically afford to significantly increase faculty compensation levels. The faculty practice plan was introduced as a way to bring more income to the faculty and to support retention and recruitment.

In 1982, a plan was developed and approved by county officials and received the support of the hospital-based faculty. There were identifiable benefits for both the county hospital and faculty members. The buy-in advantage for the county was a reduction in direct funding of faculty. The county was responsible for faculty teaching costs only, not the costs associated with professional services. The faculty buy-in advantage was the opportunity to bill patients and third parties directly for professional services and potentially increase income above the existing levels.

The faculty developed written goals to:

▲ Maintain a high-quality residency teaching program.

▲ Provide high-quality care to patients.

▲ Recruit and retain high-quality physicians.

At the time the plan was initiated, the hospital-based faculty consisted of 10 physicians. Three physicians served in a six-month pilot to test the plan before the remainder of the group entered.

## Organization and Management
*The faculty initially organized as an association and then evolved to a corporation.*

The initial organization model for the faculty was an association. This model was simple, required minimal capital from the faculty to develop, and gave the faculty an opportunity to evaluate the nature of this new business relationship with minimal risk. The faculty received the assistance of the managers of the Fresno County Hospital faculty practice plan, who developed financial pro formas, analyzed various organizational models, and recommended a model that was subsequently adopted by the faculty. Startup costs were covered from an initial contribution from each faculty member. The hospital medical director served as the association manager and chaired the weekly faculty business meetings.

In 1985, the faculty formed a partnership. The faculty needed more structure as it began to grow and perceived greater need to better manage its business and financial affairs. The partnership contracted with the hospital medical director to serve as managing partner and also with a business manager who employed two additional staff members to handle administrative and accounting services. Consequently, the partnership itself had no employees. New faculty members joined as associates and were voted into the partnership, usually after six months.

Although the association and the partnership managed faculty business, each faculty member continued to maintain individual contracts with the county. This model did not change until the faculty incorporated.

In 1992, the corporate model was developed. This final transformation occurred for several reasons. First, the faculty wanted a single contract with the county, and the corporation was the preferred contracting entity. This eliminated individual physician contracts and placed the corporation in control of the contracting process. It also made the corporation responsible for the conduct of its physicians. Second, there were tax advantages for the faculty corporation. For the first time, faculty members became employees.

At the time of incorporation, the faculty consisted of 21 primary care physicians and 7 specialists, 19 of whom were shareholders.

## Governance
*The faculty practice plan is managed by a board of directors that represents all shareholders in the corporation.*

The partnership document developed in 1985 helped tightened the legal bond of the faculty. It restated the faculty goals and defined the terms for partnership entrance and exit, the conducting of business, and the distribution of partnership income. The partnership document also included the processes for conducting business and making decisions. All resolutions and decisions require 80 percent approval of all faculty members, who are balloted in writing. Each faculty member casts one vote. Balloting is open, as each faculty member signs acceptance or rejection of a proposal on one common ballot. The goal is consensus building. This require a great deal of discussion, understanding, and harmony among faculty members. A written record of all resolutions is kept; it serves as a historic anthology of the evolution of the group. This process contributed to the organizational development of the faculty.

Upon transition to the corporation, all 19 partners became shareholders and members of the board of directors. They executed shareholder and employment agreements with the corporation. Decisions by written ballot continued. The managing partner became chief executive officer and presides over board meetings, manages the affairs of the corporation, and is empowered to make specified business decisions. This includes the authority to negotiate contracts and to make expenditures up to a specified dollar limit without board approval. A secretary-treasurer position was established as the remaining officer of the corporation.

## Practice Setting
*All faculty members have patient care as well as teaching responsibilities in the hospital and the ambulatory centers.*

The faculty provides teaching services to residents in family practice in both the hospital and the family practice center. In addition, each primary care faculty member has a panel of private patients. Most of the family practice faculty members provide obstetrical services. Call schedules were established to cover all inpatient services. Community-based faculty members under contract with the medical group provide subspecialty coverage and supplement the teaching of residents.

## Revenue and Expense Distributions
*Faculty revenue is derived from teaching and professional services. Income and expenses are allocated by an agreed-upon formula.*

Until 1992, each faculty member was paid by the county for teaching services on an hourly rate. Each faculty member negotiated a maximum number of allowable hours that could be billed in a pay period. When the faculty incorporated in 1992, the corporation negotiated one price with the county for all teaching services based on an analysis of total teaching hours needed. This was determined by the director of the family practice residency and the service chiefs. The teaching hours were then apportioned to each faculty member following individual negotiations with the residency director and the service chiefs. The faculty employment agreements addressed salary and professional requirements.

The faculty pays rent to the hospital for office space for medical services in the ambulatory sites. The hospital's malpractice carrier provided a rider to include faculty teaching and non-teaching components. These costs are reimbursed to the hospital.

Corporate expenses are not limited to but include all faculty salaries, compensation of the chief executive officer and the group manager, rent, secretarial and accounting support, billing fees, malpractice, medical expenses, legal services, business supplies and equipment, travel, retirement plan contributions, and educational and retreat expenses. All nonphysician staff members remain employees of the hospital and are not a direct expense to the faculty plan. The faculty contracts with a professional billing service that bills and collects for all patient care services.

## Faculty Compensation

Faculty salaries are derived from teaching and direct patient care. Teaching income is fixed, based on previously described negotiations. The corporation retains 5 percent of total patient care income for a profitsharing fund. The fund was established as a means of supplementing the income of primarily "administrative" physicians and nonprocedure-oriented specialists. The remaining 95 percent, after expenses, is distributed in proportion to individual collections. Profit-sharing income is distributed equally. For example, Dr. A's salary in a given month might be $7,600, derived as follows:

| | | |
|---|---|---|
| Teaching | | $3,000.00 |
| Gross patient income | $5,236.84 | |
| Allocated expenses | -1,552.63 | |
| Net patient care | $3,684.21 | |
| | | |
| 95% of patient care | | $3,500.00 |
| Profit sharing | | $1,100.00* |
| Total income | | $7,600.00 |

* Represents 5% of total patient care income of the corporation, minus expenses, divided by the number of faculty participants.

Salaries vary from month to month as patient care income varies.

## Successes and Failures

*The faculty practice plan positively influences the hospital, the residency program, and the community.*

The faculty practice plan is a success, as evidenced by the low faculty turnover and success in recruiting both faculty and outstanding residents in family practice. Salary levels are competitive and contribute positively to low turnover. From 1982 to 1992, the faculty group increased from 10 to 28 physicians. During that same period, only six physicians left the group, primarily because of career opportunities. One became a residency director, another the director of a university-based family practice network. The residency has always matched among its top choices in the National Residency Matching Program; the reputation of the faculty is a contributing factor in this achievement.

The consensus process of decision making by the faculty has led to a high degree of camaraderie. This camaraderie extends to the families of faculty members, especially during semi-annual retreats held at nearby resorts. The retreats provide both a business and a very valuable social function. Faculty members have a high level of job satisfaction.

The faculty makes good business financial plans. An example is the prefunding of retreat expenses over the course of the year. This avoids single large cash outlays from group income. In addition, the faculty created a research and development) account, funded from monthly earnings. This account is used to support major activities of the hospital and residency program. It also serves as an emergency source of faculty income during a cashflow crisis.

In 1986, the hospital was threatened with closure, and the faculty agreed to reduce teaching fees to support the hospital.[3] The faculty rallied again in 1989 during another fiscal crisis and agreed to assist the county in supplementing the salary of a new hospital chief executive officer.

The faculty provides support for many community not-for-profit activities, residency social activities, residency expansion, residency emergency loans, and employee recognition activities.

*Very few aspects of the faculty practice plan pose real and/or potential problems.*

There is no cap on practice income. For a few providers, this causes a conflict between teaching time and patient care, where the greater incentive is to provide patient care. The lack of a cap also leads to disparate incomes between primary care providers and the higher paid procedure-oriented faculty. The procedure-oriented specialists periodically raise concerns about their proportionally higher contributions to the profit-sharing plan. However, this has not become a divisive issue.

The group allows individual faculty members on a case-by-case basis to practice part time in the community. This policy creates conflicts in their availability for teaching and/or faculty practice activities, but the practice continues.

## Summary

*The faculty practice plan has achieved its goals.*

The faculty practice plan in Modesto, California, has developed into a successful model at a public teaching hospital. The faculty evolved from an association to a corporation over a 10-year span. Group camaraderie, salary levels, and a sense of job satisfaction contribute to faculty growth and retention and to a highly regarded residency program.

## References

1. Schmidt, C., and others. "A Practice Plan in a Municipal Teaching Hospital: A Model for the Funding of Clinical Faculty." *New England Journal of Medicine* 304(5):263-9, Jan. 29, 1981.

2. Goldman, A., and Hendrix, O. "Developing Practice Plans in a Public Hospital." *Medical Group Management Journal* 32(1):64-7, Jan.-Feb. 1985.

3. Boddie, W., and others. "Financial Crisis in a Family Practice Residency: A Successful Strategy." *Journal of Family Practice* 29(2):201-4, Aug. 1989.

*William L. Boddie, MD, is currently Associate Medical Director for Business Affairs, Southeast Permanent Medical Group, Atlanta, Ga. He formerly served as President and Chief Executive Officer, Scenic Faculty Medical Group, and Medical Director, Stanislaus Medical Center.*

# Chapter 7

▲  ▲  ▲

## Department Practice Plan to Respond to Managed Care Environment

by Gene F. Conway, MD, John Dorfmeister, MA,
and Robert G. Luke, MD

We will discuss in this chapter the current University Internal Medicine Associates (UIMA) Practice Plan at the University of Cincinnati Medical Center and then provide a description of a modified practice plan that is being developed as a model for use during transition of the UIMA practice to one in which compensation is significantly or predominantly affected by capitated or contracted programs. We postulate that, within the next two to five years, the Cincinnati market will be significantly capitated and/or under contracted care (40-60 percent of total revenues). The penetration could be larger, depending on the speed and effectiveness with which Medicare reimbursement is shifted to a managed care model. We anticipate that no more than 10-15 percent of the market will remain indemnity care.

The current practice plan is heavily incentive-driven and was implemented approximately eight years ago, at a time when our payer mix was 40 percent private insurance, 30 percent Medicare, and 15 percent Medicaid, with the remainder being largely self-pay. This payer mix remained essentially the same until about two years ago, with a subsequent decrease of approximately 10 percent in the private insurance component that has been partly replaced (less than 5 percent) by managed care, which is largely capitated. The practice plan has been quite successful, showing a 400 percent increase in clinical productivity (billings/collections) over the past six years.

The modified plan differs from the current practice plan principally by introducing significant changes in the method of compensating clinicians. These changes are intended to encourage practice behavior that we anticipate will be necessary for success under capitated or contracted compensation. We recognize that the proposed additional steps involved in physician compensation represent a significant increase in the administrative burden of the practice plan. However, this should be manageable, because the required data input will have to be collected by the group practice in order to successfully manage physician compensation, as well as to control practice patterns under managed and contracted care.

---

## Clinical Practice Plan.

### General Goals

Current
▲ Encourage faculty productivity
▲ Decentralize management and fiscal responsibilities

Proposed
▲ Encourage faculty productivity as a function of service and cost-effective practices
▲ Establish management and fiscal basis for integration into group practice

### Physician Compensation

Current
▲ Function of episodes of care and procedures in FFS environment

Proposed
▲ Function of patient service and satisfaction, case management and outcomes, efficient and economic use of resources

---

The current faculty practice plan is essentially a decentralized model, with a high degree of individual department autonomy, but we have begun to move to an increasing level of coordination, with increasing elements of common governance among department practices. We expect to move to a group model, with common governance and central administration.

Ultimately, we envision an equity-model multispecialty group practice that will operate as a private multispecialty group practice. Physicians will be salaried at competitive rates, with their services reimbursed through academic clinical departments. Practice income will serve as a variable but significant percentage of total compensation for each physician. The group practice will manage all clinical practices, will pay practice plan costs, and will produce a surplus that will be used to support department academic efforts and eliminate the need for much of the current taxation model.

# Current Practice Plan

### Objectives of the Practice Plan

The objectives of the current practice plan are to:

▲ Ensure fairness and consistency, comprehensibility, and reward of productivity and merit in the areas of patient care, teaching, and research.

▲ Stabilize divisional budgets, which include most of the income and most of the expenditures relevant to the faculty and the division. Both income and spending will be controlled where they can best be monitored.

▲ Recognize that industrial (contract) studies will continue to grow and that faculty must include a fair component of salary in their costs and budgets.

## Oversight and Management

The practice plan must conform with the principles and guidelines of the University of Cincinnati College of Medicine group practice plan and be approved by the Dean of the College of Medicine. The plan is governed by the Departmental Practice Plan Advisory Committee, which is composed of four faculty members who are actively practicing clinicians and is chaired by the Director of the Department. The Practice Plan Advisory Committee approves and/or develops policy for the plan, oversees plan administration, and approves and/or makes fiscal policy.

Day-to-day management of the business functions of the practice plan is under the direction of the department's business director. The various division directors are responsible for the clinical activities of the department, both inpatient and ambulatory. The Associate Director for Clinical Affairs works with the division directors and individual faculty physicians to integrate and facilitate practice activities.

The Departmental Medical Practice Committee is advisory to the practice plan regarding fee schedules, practice policies, managed care plans, and operation of the faculty ambulatory practice, as well as business functions that affect the faculty's clinical practice.

## Fiscal Plan

### Revenues

All cash collections deriving from all physician professional services are credited to the physicians rendering the service. Practice costs are allocated to all physician services except for discounted fees from government payers that may accrue at some sites of service. Fifty percent of outpatient laboratory surpluses in private patient settings are allocated to the respective divisions on behalf of their attending physicians on a per visit basis. It is understood that these revenues are not derived in any part from payment by government payers.

Income from external contracts for patient care responsibilities are allocated as follows:

| Department | 5 percent |
|---|---|
| Division | 5 percent |
| Individuals | 90 percent |

Clinical trials and other external contracts for clinical research or other services of faculty physicians are budgeted as follows:

5 percent for departmental business expenses
2 percent for group practice expenses
93 percent to the division:

— 10 percent for time and effort of principal investigator
— 10 percent for divisional costs
— Balance for clinical trial expenses

Any surplus remaining at the conclusion of a project is distributed as agreed upon by the division director and the faculty principal investigator (PI).

Sales and services of laboratory or other division business activities are to be handled within University and Corporate policies. The Department is allocated 5 percent of collections for business, finance, and administrative costs associated with the activities.

Research Incentive Award (RIA) earnings represent an arbitrary fraction of research or contract overhead paid to the parent university that is returned to the department and division holding the primary contract or award. RIA funds are allocated from both federal and private sources that pay indirect costs. These earnings can be used at the discretion of the division director and the PI. RIA is allocated 60 percent to the division and 40 percent to the department.

Division base support is derived from a combination of state general funds, Medicare Part "A" funds, general endowments, and clinical teaching subsidies. Divisions with deficits are severely restricted in their ability to provide discretionary spending for academic support for journals, travel, etc.

### Costs
Faculty compensation (salaries and benefits) are a divisional expense. Wages and benefits of all support and ancillary personnel are a divisional expense. Costs of all supplies, stationery, phones, travel, etc. supporting divisional/faculty activity are divisional expenses. Clinical trial expenses are to be paid from divisional trial cash receipts. Direct corporation expenses are charged to appropriate trial corporate accounts. If College of Medicine resources are used, the college is reimbursed by the practice corporation. Expenses for grants and other financed research activities are charged to the specific restricted grant accounts.

Costs are allocated to fee for service (FFS) collections from professional services as follows:

| | |
|---|---|
| Practice Support | 16 percent |
| Billing | 10 percent |
| Department Share | 10 percent |
| Division Share | 10 percent |
| Professional Liability | 2 percent |
| Group Practice | 2 percent |

The remaining 50 percent is attributed to the divisions for the individuals rendering the services. For the practice track (see below), the 50 percent allocation is credited to the individual faculty member for salary and fringe benefits.

*Faculty Compensation*

Faculty are compensated according to guidelines developed for three tracks that are not necessarily equivalent to the academic tracks of the college:

▲ **Leadership Track**—for division directors and administrative positions within the department. Compensation for these individuals is determined in consideration of both internal and external factors and in consideration of their individual performance and the overall performance of the functional entity for which they are responsible.

▲ **Clinical/Investigator/Educator Track**—faculty members in this track are given a target percentage (agreed upon by individual, division director, and department chair) of proposed annual salary and fringe benefits to bring in from all sources. Any monies brought in by faculty members' efforts for personal salary above the target are divided as follows:

— One-third individual (or for personal academic purposes) distributed at the end of year. This amount can be distributed as additional salary and benefits.

— One-third division.

— One-third department.

Stable increases in income may be included in salary in subsequent years.

▲ **Practice Track**—This track is entered upon only by agreement of the individual, the division director, and the department chair. It is designed for faculty members whose primary responsibility is to build and maintain practices. The faculty will receive a base salary from division funds (which include the divisional base support) and may receive compensation for designated activities (e.g., teaching), bonus income, or other clinically derived compensation as discussed later.

## The Proposed Faculty Practice Plan

Much of the existing practice plan structures and policies, as outlined above, will be unchanged. However, significant changes in the compensation of physician members of the plan are contemplated in order to make incentives more conducive to a managed care, capitated environment.

### Objectives of the Proposed Practice Plan

The objectives of the proposed practice plan are to:

▲ Serve as a transition vehicle for business functions and management of the faculty practice plan to adapt to participation and contract into managed care.

▲ Align compensation of faculty clinicians with changing patterns of compensation for health care deriving from contracts in managed care and encourage collegiality and team behaviors.

▲ Ensure a continuing source of revenue to support the academic programs of the Department of Internal Medicine and the College of Medicine.

▲ Provide for the availability of patients to support education and research.

▲ Encourage superior patient care, teaching, and research.

## Fiscal Plan

### *Revenues*

During the transitional period, all cash collections derived from physicians' professional services will continue to be credited to the physicians rendering the services. Revenues from outpatient laboratory services in private patient settings have decreased rapidly and, for all practical purposes, have ceased to be a factor in faculty compensation. At low fractions (less than 20 percent) of capitated and contracted care, revenue derived from these services will be credited to the physicians rendering the services, with practice costs allocated as above but with reduction of 10 percent percent for billing costs to 5 percent to cover bookkeeping and administrative costs, thus increasing to 55 percent the amount credited for salary and fringe benefits. However, cost accounting procedures are being devised to more accurately allocate support costs for programs and practice activities. The revised cost accounting procedures will also support negotiation for adequate captitation fees and contracts for care of a defined population. As managed care evolves, cost accounting will become a continuous process.

### *Compensation of Clinical Faculty*

During the transitional period, FFS and other compensation techniques not governed by managed care organizations (MCOs) or contracts will continue to be distributed according to existing productivity guidelines (e.g., 50 percent of collections are applied to salary targets or bonus payments).

Distribution of surplus dollars from contract and compensation from MCOs will be governed by the guidelines given below. Returned withholds will be applied to a primary care "risk" pool. Pools will be set up with surplus distribution as follows:

▲ Primary Care: Surplus to Primary Care Physicians' bonus pool

▲ Specialty Care: Surplus to Specialty Physicians bonus pool

▲ Hospital: Surplus distributed to Primary Care and to Specialty Physicians bonus pools with allocations based on realized savings by each group

### *Primary Care Compensation*

The base amount of compensation will be the negotiated fixed annual salary with productivity target (availability and productivity, e.g., patient encounters). Eligibility for bonus will depend on exceeding the target. The amount of compensation provided for teaching activities will be fixed through negotiation and will be based on total teaching efforts. A teaching "practice plan" has been devised and implemented, which permits objective quantification of the teaching effort of individual faculty.* A primary care physician's bonus pool will be constituted as indicated above. The total available pool will be assigned for distribution according to the percentages shown below. Each primary care physician's bonus will be calculated as described in the appendix to this chapter and will be based on the individual's performance in each of the categories below.

Any undistributed funds will be retained on the basis of 50 percent in the bonus pool and 50 percent for distribution from the "risk" pool.

▲ Productivity: 35 percent of the pool: will be based on units of service (hospital and out-patient visits, capitated or contracted procedures).

▲ Cost per ambulatory patient visit: 30 percent of the pool.

▲ Utilization of special referrals inside and outside the group: 15 percent of the pool.

▲ Patient services (quality assurance and patient surveys): 10 percent of the pool.

▲ Case management (outcomes, hospital length of stays, hospital days/1000, preventive care): 10 percent of the pool.

\* Rouan, G., and others. "Utilizing a Practice Plan to Reimburse Faculty Effort in the Teaching of Medical Students and House Staff." In preparation for publication.

Funds, up to 50 percent of the bonus pool, will be withheld for one year and distributed when group objectives are met. The pool will benefit from return of withholds from MCOs and from any surpluses that may be realized from primary care, specialty care, and hospital pools.

Among the criteria used for distribution of funds from the pools to the physicians are:

▲ Meeting financial goals.

▲ Meeting referral targets.

▲ Meeting targets for use of laboratory and other tests.

▲ Percentage of contract or capitated patients cared for by physician.

### Specialty Care Compensation
Compensation of specialty care physicians will be based on the current productivity model for indemnity-type FFS care. Discounted FFS payment or subcapitation will be used for specialty physicians under managed care contracts, and subcapitation will be used for specialty physicians under capitation contracts.

Bonuses to subspecialty providers will be considered if there is a surplus in the specialists' pool (also receives contribution from any surplus in hospital pool) for capitated and con-tracted care. Among the criteria for distribution of specialists' bonus pool funds are:

▲ Outcomes indicators: readmissions, repeat procedures, adverse reactions or outcomes, and of functional patients.

▲ Patient satisfaction

## Appendix: Calculation of Physician Bonus for Capitated and Contracted Care Compensation

▲ *Productivity (35% of Pool $)*
   *Bonus = (0.35)(A)(B)(C)*

Where:          A = Total Pool $

                B = Physician's units of service
                    Group total units of service

                C = Physician's units of service
                    Target units of service

▲ *Cost per Ambulatory Visit (30% of Pool $)*
   *Bonus = (0.30)(A)(D)(E)*

Where:          A = Total Pool $

                D = Physician's ambulatory visits
                    Group total ambulatory visits

                E = Group's average visit cost – Physician's average visit cost
                    Group's average visit cost

▲ *Referral Utilization (15% of Pool $)*
   *Bonus = (0.15)(A)(D)(F)*

Where:          A = Total Pool $

                D = Physician's ambulatory visits
                    Group's total ambulatory visits

                F = Group's average (or target) referral – Physician's referrals
                    Group average (or target) referrals

▲ *Patient Service (10% of Pool $)*
   *Bonus = (0.10)(A)(D)(I)*

Where:          A = Total Pool $

                D = $\dfrac{\text{Physician's ambulatory visits}}{\text{Group total ambulatory visits}}$

                I = $\dfrac{\text{Physician's score on target}}{\text{Group average score on target}}$

Target here represents achievement of goals for patient satisfaction.

▲ *Case Management (10% of Pool $)*
   *Bonus = (0.10)(A)(G)(H)*

Where:          A = Total Pool $

                G = $\dfrac{\text{Number of panel patients}}{\text{Group's total panel patients}}$

                H = $\dfrac{\text{Physician's score on target}}{\text{Group's average score on target}}$

Target is a composite of targets for achievement on outcomes, hospital length of stay, hospital days/1,000, and specified items of preventive care.

---

*Gene F. Conway, MD, is Professor of Medicine and Associate Chairman, Department of Internal Medicine, College of Medicine, University of Cincinnati Medical Center, Cincinnati, Ohio. John Dorfmeister, MA, is Executive Director of University Internal Medicine Associates, Cincinnati, and Robert G. Luke, MD, is Chairman, Department of Internal Medicine, College of Medicine, University of Cincinnati Medical Center.*

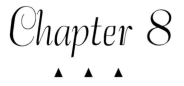

# Chapter 8

▲  ▲  ▲

## Establishing a Centralized Faculty Practice Plan

by Martin S. Litwin, MD

$\mathcal{C}$learly, faculty practice plan (FPP) revenues are increasingly important in the financial structure of academic health centers. Funds generated by clinicians from professional fees for patient care are now indispensable to support medical education.[1] It is for this reason that there is widespread interest in the clinical practices of faculty members. Practice plans developed as a result of the foresight of those who recognized that practice revenues would become important to academic health centers as other revenue sources became weaker. Early practice plans were usually department- or section-based. Schoolwide or hospitalwide centralized practice plans evolved somewhat later. These are characterized by centralized governance, billing, collections and record keeping.[2] In this chapter, methods will be presented for establishing centralized practice plan authority, the preferable methods for maintaining central FPP control will be described, and the advantages of a central FPP structure will be detailed.

## FPP Agreement
Establishment of a centralized FPP requires the development of written rules and regulations.[2] An outline for a centralized practice plan agreement is shown at the end of this chapter in Appendix A, page 63-64. An FPP constitution and bylaws or FPP agreement is of benefit both to the group as a whole and to each FPP member. A clear statement of purpose, definition of levels and requirements of membership, and rules for regulation and implementation of principles defined by the FPP governing body ensures compliance by participating practice plan members and defines the relationship of the FPP to other organizations and boards to which its members may be responsible.

## Governance and Representation
A controversial problem in establishing a centralized FPP is determining an appropriate method for deciding equitable representation on the FPP governing body. This is one of the first provisions that should be developed and included in the formal FPP agreement. Members of departments that have large numbers of participants who generate lower levels of income may perceive that, because there are larger numbers of participants within their department, they should have larger representation and greater voice in the governance of the FPP. Those who come from smaller departments that generate higher levels of

income may expect that their representation in governance of the practice plan should be greater, especially when a portion of their revenues is used to subsidize overhead in departments that generate less revenue. An astute physician executive can easily see that all these participants are necessary for the success of a centralized FPP and that the interests of all must be considered and protected. This can be accomplished most equitably by giving equal recognition to the total number of physicians within a department and to total revenue generated by the department.

Using this method, a section of primary care medicine with 20 physicians who generate $4,000,000 in total revenues per year would achieve equitable representation with an eight-man department of orthopedics that generates a total of $10,000,000 in the same period. However, every department, even the smallest, must have at least one representative. The method to calculate representation is described in Appendix B, page 65.

Until a method for deciding equitable representation is agreed upon by all FPP participants, it is not possible to achieve satisfactory FPP centralization. This issue may be so divisive that it becomes a destructive force if an attempt is made to deal with it in an authoritarian fashion. A high level of agreement and cooperation is required for the success of any centralized FPP. For this reason, election of members from each department is clearly the preferred method for constituting the FPP governing body. Empowerment of a department's representatives is most firm when they are elected democratically. Autocratic appointment of the FPP governing body is possible, but widespread unhappiness and disagreement, administrative distrust, and passive uncooperation will usually follow. Democratic principles allow a centralized group to become a functioning and effective one much more quickly than is the case when an autocratic appointment method is used.

Because the business of the FPP frequently involves past events, it is advantageous to retain a degree of institutional and/or program memory among the members of the FPP governing body. Members should be elected for a term long enough to allow well-thought-out policy decisions to be made and programs to be enacted. In general the optimal interval for elections appears to be every two years. At the end of two years, calculations should again be done to make certain that equitable representation is maintained on the basis of both numbers of department participants and levels of revenue generated. New elections are then carried out, and a new governing body is empowered. Reelection of members who have served satisfactorily during the preceding two years contributes to the institutional memory mentioned earlier.

## Credentialing

In an academic setting, FPP professional credentialing is done in association with the faculty appointment process by the dean's office, working in conjunction with the personnel and honors committee. Procedures followed are the same whether the FPP is centralized or department-based and are similar to those necessary to secure a hospital staff appointment. These procedures include verification of medical school graduation and state licensure, National Practioner Data Bank inquiries, information from state medical societies and other medical schools and hospitals at which the individual may have held previous appointments, etc.

Usually, credentialing for hospital privileges must be accomplished through the hospital medical staff office separately from the FPP appointment process. Even though a physician may have been approved for a medical school appointment, regulations of the Joint Commission on Accreditation of Healthcare Organizations require that the physician be independently credentialed within the hospital according to procedures outlined in the hospital by-laws.

## Taxation and Income Distribution

Of paramount importance are clearly worded, well-defined regulations in the FPP agreement for the generation and distribution of income. This minimizes potential conflict and also contractually protects the entire FPP against litigation that may arise from disgruntled FPP members. The method by which FPP group cost of practice or overhead is paid and individual compensation is determined is a potentially explosive and contentious issue that any centralized FPP must face. This should also be clearly defined. In order to achieve equity, all funds derived from all professional activities of all FPP members should be credited to individual faculty members and be used as one factor in determining individual salary or income. Frequently, FPP members will feel that monies derived from certain types of professional activities in which they engage should either not be reported or not be turned in as required. Others may feel that their activities should be taxed or assessed at a lesser rate than the rate defined in the FPP agreement.

For example, arguments will be made that monies derived by primary care physicians from capitation contracts or by plastic surgeons from payment in advance for cosmetic procedures should be taxed at a lesser rate. A typical rationalization is that such revenues do not require billing and collection procedures; hence, the support of administrative personnel usually involved in these activities is not necessary. It is for this reason that the terms for cost-of-practice assessment on all professional income must be clearly spelled out in the FPP agreement. All regulations relating to other assessments, such as dean's and departmental taxes, and to distribution of revenues derived from sources other than patient care must also be very clearly stated. To ensure compliance with financial regulations in the FPP agreement that require reporting of all income, each FPP member should be required to submit a year-end federal tax return to the Medical Director or the FPP Administrator for confidential review. The lack of full compliance by all FPP members with regulations governing professional income must be dealt with by the FPP governing body firmly and in a reasonable and consistent fashion. Noncompliance by any FPP member can ultimately lead to financial embarrassment for and disintegration of the entire organization.

## Medical Director and FPP Administrator

The only permanent member of the FPP governing body is the Medical Director, who should be chair. It is beyond the scope of this chapter to describe the personality and other attributes necessary in a successful Medical Director; however, the Medical Director is the focal point for all of the professional activities of the FPP. It is his or her responsibility to monitor and broadly direct clinical programs; to protect the interests of individual members of the practice plan; and to mediate disputes that invariably arise between physicians. A Medical Director who consistently is aligned with any practice plan faction cannot be successful. Consistent alignment with a single group or individual, especially one whose interests are self-serving, will quickly alienate the Medical Director from those who have empowered him or her. The Medical Director's guiding principle must be broad institutional interests, whether leading a group practice or a hospital/group affiliation. His or her vision must ensure that the broadest possible group interests are served.

In general, the Medical Director is responsible to the FPP governing body, which is responsible for making both professional and administrative policies. The Medical Director oversees the implementation and enforcement of these policies and ensures conformity with all FPP rules. In general, the environment, organization, professional staff, financial requirements, and policy issues of the FPP are all the responsibility of the Medical Director and the governing body. Committees of the FPP governing body should also oversee billing and collections, budget and finance, and clinic operations.

A senior practice plan manager or administrator is also required for direct line implementation of all administrative aspects of a centralized FPP. This administrator has the responsibility to implement and enforce FPP administrative and business policies set by the governing body and to ensure effective day-to-day operations of the practice plan. Clinic operation, business office oversight, budget preparation, and a host of other administrative functions require that this FPP manager be a trained health care administrator. Again, it is beyond the scope of this chapter to discuss the qualities necessary in a successful FPP administrator. Institutional loyalty, appropriate administrative knowledge, and an ability and desire to understand and relate to the needs of practicing physicians are all necessary attributes.

## Peer Review

A centralized faculty practice facilitates ongoing review of physician behavior and practice patterns in both offfice and hospital setting. Peer review in a centralized practice plan can lead to considerably more effective medical service utilization, more effficient practice patterns, delivery of better quality health care, and higher levels of patient satisfaction than might be possible in separate department or section practice plans. All of these parameters are of importance to managed care organizations and are equally important to the financial well-being of the FPP, especially when dealing with patients under capitated agreement.

When peer review is done within the FPP, the Medical Director must make certain that the reviews are objective and honest. If peer reviewers have unrelated personal or vested interests, great harm to the entire group can result. Ensuring objective peer review is an important responsibility of the Medical Director.

No matter what the financial circumstances, the group collectively and the Medical Director individually must make certain that each physician's fiduciary responsibility to each patient is not compromised. Incident reports, letters and telephone calls from patients, and verbal and written reports from employees working in all sections of the FPP often serve to lead to those areas that may be potentially problematic.

Even though somewhat outside the realm of peer review, "Standards of Service" will be of use. These FPP regulations define administrative standards to which all FPP members are expected to adhere. The central FPP governing body should assist in the development of such standards and approve them. A regular reporting mechanism should be implemented, and the Medical Director should review physician/patient, physician/staff, and staff/patient interactions on a regular basis.

All breaches of quality of care, as perceived either by patients or by other physicians, must come to the attention of the Medical Director. The department chairs are responsible for ensuring that actual breaches in quality of care do not recur. If the offending physician is a department chair or if the department chair does not take corrective action, the Medical Director must deal with such problems quickly and firmly.

Quality issues are frequently the basis for malpractice suits. Whether such suits are found to be justified or unjustified, they can destroy both the reputation and the financial integrity of the group. For this reason, appropriate legal counsel in health law must be readily available when needed. A respected, competent, and sophisticated attorney can often assist greatly in avoiding or minimizing contentious situations that may expose the group to liability.

## Accountability

In a centralized FPP, financial accountability is difficult to achieve unless very specific regulations are developed. A uniform cost-of-practice assessment spread across all members of the practice plan will be unsuccessful if practice plan members do not treat overhead costs paid from a central fund as conservatively as when such costs are accounted for and paid individually. Financial accountability can be partially successful if very strict budgetary guidelines are developed and enforced, but it has been the author's experience that colleagues find it extraordinarily difficult to deny colleagues' requests for expenditures of funds. Even when the expenditure requested is a variance from budget, it will invariably be permitted unless there are explicit written policies in the FPP agreement prohibiting expenditures outside the budget. The latter rarely are written as explicitly as may be required in dealing with a contentious and determined FPP member.

A method that ensures accountability and frugality is one in which a specific dollar amount is allocated by the FPP governing body to each department or cost center. Justified and reasonable expenditures during a previous period can serve as the basis for determining the amount of this allocation. The group should feel the base dollar amount is adequate for support of the particular section or division of the practice. Financial requirements of a cost center above the amount allocated and budgeted should be the responsibility of the department in which the cost center is located. Budgeted funds not expended by the cost center to which the allocation is made can then revert at year-end to practitioners. This provides an excellent incentive to conserve funds and is essentially the same method as that used by HMOs in the capitation process.

## Billing and Collection Procedures

Another activity that clearly distinguishes a centralized practice plan from a decentralized one is billing and collection. The difficulties in implementing and participating in a centralized system when multiple smaller and simpler department or section billing systems exist are manifold; however, if the FPP expects to negotiate and develop affiliations with large insurance carriers and managed care organizations, a centralized billing system is mandatory. It permits all charges from all departments to be entered on a singled itemized bill by a data processing office acting through the central billing office. Each patient receives one bill for all professional services. All charges, payments, insurance billings, and amounts due should be clearly shown. A centralized billing system also permits close follow-up of outstanding accounts and collection activities on behalf of all members of the practice plan that would not otherwise be possible.

Most patients are very naive in matters relating to health insurance coverage. Many who are not naive frequently will profess to be so in an attempt to avoid paying their bills. A single, itemized, fully explained statement that shows all insurance billings, payments, discounts, and personal balances is difficult to contest and will minimize this problem. Several computer systems that permit generation of such a bill already exist. Because of increasing demand, other such systems may be expected to be developed in the next several years.

## Billing, Documentation, and Compliance

A centralized billing system and a single central billing office have become increasingly important as more rigid enforcement of federal statutes related to professional billing and reimbursement have been developed. The Stark Laws, other health care fraud and abuse statutes, and Health Care Financing Administration (HCFA) regulations are now extraordinarily important in professional billing. A centralized practice plan billing process allows more careful supervision to prevent violations of all legally mandated billing requirements. Because of heavy financial penalties and possible criminal prosecution allowed under the law, the integrity of the group practice can be endangered when billing violations are found. Even when no violation is found, financial liability incurred for audit and legal expenses can be extraordinarily large. Suffice it to say that, before a bill for professional services is rendered, there must be adequate written documentation in the patient record to justify that the charges submitted are at the correct levels, that there has been no up-coding and/or charge unbundling, and that the bill has been prepared in the names of the physicians who rendered the services.

At the time of this writing, the U.S. Department of Health and Human Services' Office of Inspector General has undertaken a nationwide review of compliance with rules governing physicians at teaching hospitals and with other Medicare payment rules. HCFA also recently published in the *Federal Register* a strict interpretation of IL-372 that is related to billing for professional services rendered to Medicare and Medicaid recipients in an academic teaching center.

Although this chapter will not discuss the many facets of professional billing, recognition of legal billing requirements is mandatory both in the FPP Agreement and individually by each member of the FPP who submits bills for patient care services. This can best be accomplished when using a centralized billing system. Appendix C, page 66, outlines a compliance program that is felt by the author to be of use in complying with Medicare billing regulations.

## Departmental Modifications

Allowances can be made in the FPP agreement for departmental differences in practice patterns and types of practices, even though FPP administration may be highly centralized and the FPP centrally governed. One department may wish to devote more time to charity practice, research, or teaching, while another may wish to concentrate on clinical practice and generation of income. Still others may have contracts or grants allowing them to perform highly specialized care or clinical research. The role of the department chair in determining type and intensity of work parameters and income distribution may also vary, depending on the wishes of FPP members in the department. As long as a department abides by the general principles in the centralized FPP agreement, there is no reason that practice patterns and the method for work load and income distribution cannot vary according to the needs and desires of the FPP members in that department. When a department institutes programs and principles that are at variance with the general FPP agreement, conflict results within the department. It is the responsibility of the Medical Director to ensure equitable treatment for all members of the FPP, even when a decision is at variance with the desires of others in the department.

## Termination

Even in the most equitable and generous faculty practice plans, member resignations will occur. General business contractual principles, geographic covenants, and practice restrictions must be in place to protect the FPP. Otherwise, terminations can be very damaging. There should be clear provisions in the FPP agreement indicating that, when separation occurs, all patient records remain the property of the practice plan. Lack of this regulation will allow disgruntled FPP members to leave the practice with information on significant numbers of patients who have been cared for by the FPP. Clear-cut regulations in the FPP agreement will minimize this risk and provide legal protection against it.

Provisions should also be included in the FPP agreement for appropriate handling of all accounts receivable of a departing physician. In general, it is equitable to handle accounts receivable during the first 12 months after the faculty member's departure in the same fashion that they were handled before the departure. Unless there has been a deficit in the departing member's, payments based on these earnings should be continued. After 12 months, it is reasonable to expect that any remaining accounts receivable will revert to the entire group.

## Advantages

Managed care and increasingly restrictive reimbursement guidelines offer both opportunities and threats to all group practices, especially to those associated with faculty practice plans. In financial and business circles, centrally controlled plans with uniform policies applied across all departments are viewed with considerably more favor than are those with a strong emphasis on individual sections and departments.[3] A centralized FPP will probably find it considerably easier than a department plan to enter financial markets for borrowing or for other forms of capitalization. Centralization of FPP governance also prevents departmental duplication of expensive services (billing, collection, purchasing, etc.) and activities (total quality management, outcomes analysis, cost control, etc.).

Implicit in FPP centralization is the presence of a single, centrally empowered entity to carry on the business of the plan. Managed care contracting can also be negotiated best through a central authority. Administrators of managed care companies simply will not go from department to department within a medical center and negotiate separately. Time constraints and the high level of business sophistication required also make it decidedly advantageous to the individual FPP physicians to have their represented by a trusted small group. In a centralized FPP, a small group can be empowered to represent the entire practice plan and to negotiate on its behalf not only outside but also inside the institution. The FPP usually has large numbers of employees, so centralized human resource management assures conformity with multiple government regulations. When work supervision is centralized, with a clear chain of command, there is considerably less conflict and more satisfactory oversight of employees.

## Disadvantages

Effective implementation of a centralized FPP requires a degree of trust and cooperation among the FPP members that invariably is difficult to achieve, particularly at the outset. Department practice plans have considerably fewer members. Each member feels a significantly greater sense of authority and responsibility for his or her practice than is the case in a centralized FPP. Usually, a department practice plan will be governed by the department chair. The chair may rule in an autocratic fashion, but his or her interests relating to practice are usually consonant with those of department members.

In a department system, each faculty member will feel closer to his or her practice and more responsible for it; however, income distribution under such a system often leads to unhappiness and dissatisfaction, especially among members generating the largest amounts of revenue. Even though a centralized billing system and generation of a single bill for multiple services is desirable, physicians feel more comfortable when they are closer to the billing and collection portion of their practices than is possible in a large centralized FPP. Many may feel that their individual accounts are not correctly and aggressively pursued and that collection of their charges would be better accomplished at a department level. Perceived incorrect billing and inadequate accounts collection is probably the single most common argument given for a departmentalized FPP rather than a centralized one.

## Lessons from the Past

At the Tulane University Medical School, several departments had separate faculty practice plans prior to 1975. In 1975, the Medical Center Board of Governors and the Dean mandated the formation of a centralized, schoolwide FPP, with required participation by all full-time faculty in clinical departments. The original FPP agreement was written and the FPP was democratically constituted by a group of faculty after the mandate from the Dean. The original FPP members also appointed the Medical Director, who served as chair of the FPP governing body. During the first FPP organizing meetings, the FPP agreement was written and the FPP governing body was democratically empowered by popular vote within each department.

Initially, the governing group was concerned that participants in a faculty group practice would spend an inordinate amount of time in the practice of medicine to the exclusion of research and teaching. A ceiling on practice income was therefore imposed. Over the next several years, it became clear that this financial ceiling on income derived from clinical practice discouraged the faculty from practicing medicine. It also became clear that more practice revenues were needed by the school. FPP members agreed that it would be in their collective best interests to allow faculty to do more rather than less clinical practice. A committee was convened by the Medical Director and the FPP governing body to revise the practice income ceiling and the system of income assessment and distribution. As a result, the ceiling was removed and the modern age of centralized FPPs was entered. Surprisingly, teaching improved and research increased.

Over the next several years, clinically oriented department chairs and faculty were recruited. A committee was again convened to increase the percentage of professional revenues reverting to individual faculty members. This was done to stimulate clinical practices. This second revision was extraordinarily successful in accomplishing the desired effect.

As the FPP membership began to better understand the FPP agreement, the ingenious thought processes for which physicians are well-known became manifest. Various loopholes began to become obvious to faculty members who desired greater subsidization. The source for these funds was the central cost-of-practice fund that had been mandated for the budgeting process in the original FPP agreement.

Each year a budget was prepared by the clinic manager for the entire clinic and a cost-of-practice entry was projected. The Budget and Finance Subcommittee then reviewed, changed, and approved the budget. Throughout the budget year, the subcommittee approved expenditures from the central, departmentally uniform, cost-of-practice funds. Because of the reluctance of subcommittee members to firmly supervise expenditures by their colleagues from this central cost-of-practice fund, financial accountability was difficult to achieve, and variances from budget were allowed with increased frequency.

In about 1989, professional reimbursement began to drop because of the advent of discounted fee-for-service arrangements and the passage of the federal resource-related relative value scale system of physician payment under Medicare. Simultaneously, an increase in patient volume and the need to satisfy more and more regulations necessitated more and better computer capacity and larger numbers of administrative and business office personnel. Increasing expenses and slower increases in revenues in turn caused an increase in the FPP's cost of practice, expressed as a percentage of net collections.

A committee was constituted in 1990 to incorporate financial accountability in the FPP agreement in an attempt to control these divergent financial trends. The committee developed and recommended a budgeting system based on "base-year funding". Under this system, the FPP governing body allocates to each department for its cost of practice an amount equal to the cost of running the department's clinic during FY1990, the arbitrarily selected "base year." Each department was then mandated to decrease its cost of practice during FY1991 either by 4 percent or to 43 percent of its net revenue. The latter percentage was the overall net cost of practice on net professional collections for FY1990. Departments that decreased their cost of practice more than the required amount were allowed to retain one-fourth of the amount of their decreased costs within the department for distribution to individual physicians or in a way of their choice. The remaining three-fourths of the decreased costs was deposited into a general fund to be used for subsidization of departments whose cost of practice exceeded 43 percent of net revenues but that had succeeded in reducing their cost of practice by the mandated 4 percent. A committee composed of the Dean, the Vice

Chancellor, the Medical Director, and two members of the FPP governing body were empowered to make this latter distribution if it felt the extra funding could be justified by the department. Otherwise, the added expenses were to be taken from funds generating to the department from the FPP department assessment mandated in the FPP agreement.

Recently, another committee has been convened to decide appropriate cost-of-practice fund, Dean's Fund, and department assessments for certain new high-volume, low-reimbursement FPP revenue streams. These include funds generated in satellite clinics, monies from capitated contracts, and professional fees generated in the FPP's new primary care clinics.

It is anticipated that the concept of "base-year funding" will be continued and that financial accountability will remain a high priority. Funds remaining and accumulating in the subsidization fund will be used for implementing new programs and the development of other FPP ventures. The most important lesson that has been clearly learned is that a centralized FPP agreement must be flexible enough to allow accommodation by the FPP to changes in the health care market and in the practice of medicine. The medical director and the FPP governing body must be able to recognize the point at which changes in the FPP agreement must be made.

## Conclusions

The social and political climate in which medicine is currently practiced is fluid at best. Changes are occurring with such rapidity that it is difficult for any academic health center to adjust quickly enough. If we are to survive, mechanisms and procedures must be in place to allow exactly that. A centralized practice plan involving all clinical departments clearly presents many more advantages than do diverse departmentalized practice plans functioning independently throughout the institution. Broad acceptance, agreement, understanding, and trust are necessary for effective FPP centralization and operation.

## References

1. Bentley, J., and others. "Faculty Practice Plans: The Organization and Characteristics of Academic Medical Practice." *Academic Medicine* 66(8):433-9, Aug. 1991.

2. Krakower, J., and others. "Medical School Financing 1991-1992: Comparing Seven Different Types of Schools." *Academic Medicine* 69(1):72-81, Jan. 1994.

3. "Perspectives on Health Care Finance." Moody's Investors Service, Public Finance Department, Nov. 11, 1994, p. 4.

*Martin S. Litwin, MD, is Associate Dean and Medical Director, Faculty Practice Plan, and Robert and Viola Lobrano Professor of Surgery, Tulane University Medical Center, New Orleans, Louisiana.*

## Appendix A:  A Model for a Centralized Faculty Practice Plan Agreement

I.  Preamble

Purpose, aims, general statement of membership, and handling of income.

II.  Definitions

A. Definition of various requirements for types and levels of FPP membership, eligibility, and participation.

B. Definition of fees to be included in professional revenues, i.e., medicolegal fees, charges for various types of professional services, honoraria and royalties, etc. and statement of types of revenues that may be excluded.

C. Method for resolution of questions regarding levels of assessment and exclusion of revenues.

III.  Regulation

Methods for regulation of FPP members, appeal of decisions, and enforcement of regulations.

IV.  Income

A. Types of personal income excluded from FPP revenues.

B. Levels of various assessments, e.g., Dean's assessment, departmental assessment, fringe benefits, cost-of practice, etc.

C. Description of committee to oversee department accountability, including responsibilities, membership, meetings, methods to be used in judging qualification for subsidy, etc.

V.  Distribution of FPP funds

A. Priorities for distribution of FPP funds, including special fringe benefits package, incentives and bonuses, adjustments in cost of practice, etc.

B. Handling of individual physician contracts—methods for developing individual contracts and format to be used.

C. Definition, methods for determining, and methods for recovery of overpayment.

D. Base salary methodology.

E. Supplemental or incentive income (bonuses)—method for calculation of payments and recovering overpayment.

F. Method for generation, oversight, and expenditure of department assessments.

G. Method for generation, oversight, and expenditure of Dean's Fund assessment.

VI. Administration and governance

    A. Directions for administration of the FPP.

    B. Composition, responsibilities, and privileges of FPP Executive Committee.

    C. Composition and responsibilities of billing and collections, budget and finance, and clinic operations subcommittees.

VII. Role of department chair

Responsibility for delegating teaching and research time vs. patient care responsibilities, base salary levels, relationship with the Dean's office, etc.

VIII. Role of the medical director

Method of selecting, hiring, and discharging. Duties and responsibilities.

IX. FPP billing policy

General billing methods and policies, operational philosophy, compliance requirements, discounting policies and methods, accounting practices, professional discount policy, and exceptions to general credit and collection policies.

X. Department modifications

Statement and description of allowed departmental variations, including clear statement that adherence to FPP agreement is required.

XI. Fringe benefits

Statutory and other fringe benefits to which members of the FPP are entitled, including malpractice insurance, retirement funds, hospitalization coverage, disability insurance, life insurance, vacation, sick leave, parking privileges, sabbatical leave, etc.

XII. Revision of FPP agreement

Method by which FPP Agreement may be revised.

XIII. Termination

FPP policies for retention of patient records and accounts, withholding payments of base salary and/or bonuses, payment of final salary and incentive payments, and final audit of accounts receivable, including rights of both the institution and individual FPP members.

XIV. Resolution of disputes

Method for resolution of disputes arising with terminating FPP members relating to payments due, accounts receivable, practice covenants, etc.

## Appendix B: Calculating Equitable Representation on the FPP Governing Committee

With this method, equal emphasis is placed on the total number of FPP members within a department and on the total FPP revenue generated by that department. For example, Department A generated $4.8 million (column 2), or 8 percent of total net FPP revenues (column 4) during the fiscal year. During the same period, Department A had 18 FPP members (column 3), or 6 percent of the total number of participating faculty (column 5). The combined weight of the factors is then calculated by adding these two percentages (column 6) and dividing the sum by two (column 7). Using this method, Department A will be entitled to 7 percent of the seats on the FPP governing body. However, it is important to remember that even the smallest department should have at least one representative so that all FPP members will be represented. Calculation of representation can be done after this latter allocation has been done in order to limit the overall size of the committee.

| (1) Department Name | (2) FY Net Revenues ($millions) | (3) Number of Faculty in Department | (4) Net Revenues as % of Total | (5) Number of Faculty as % of Total | (6) Total of Column 4 and Column 5 | (7) Column 6 Percentage Divided by 2 |
|---|---|---|---|---|---|---|
| A | $4.8 | 18 | 8% | 6% | 14 | 7% |
| B | 0.8 | 7 | 1% | 2% | 3 | 2% |
| C | 0.3 | 6 | 1% | 2% | 3 | 2% |
| D | 8.9 | 76 | 15% | 24% | 39 | 20% |
| E | 1.9 | 3 | 3% | 1% | 4 | 2% |
| F | 2.1 | 14 | 4% | 4% | 8 | 4% |
| G | 4.9 | 9 | 8% | 3% | 11 | 5% |
| H | 7.8 | 11 | 13% | 4% | 17 | 9% |
| I | 1.2 | 4 | 2% | 1% | 3 | 2% |
| J | 1.4 | 16 | 2% | 5% | 7 | 4% |
| K | 6.0 | 51 | 10% | 16% | 26 | 13% |
| L | 6.1 | 53 | 11% | 17% | 28 | 12% |
| M | 3.4 | 15 | 6% | 5% | 11 | 6% |
| N | 5.8 | 25 | 10% | 8% | 18 | 9% |
| O | 2.6 | 9 | 5% | 3% | 8 | 4% |
| Total | $58.0 | 317 | | | | |

## Appendix C: Model for a Documentation Compliance Program

I. Statement that the Practice Plan's Professional Billing Compliance and Documentation Plan relates to professional fee billing and reimbursement and is in accordance with federal, state, and local laws and regulations.

II. Compliance Officer

A. List of duties and responsibilities to enhance compliance in professional fee documentation and billing;.

B. The reporting lines to be used in reporting compliance problems.

C. A statement of the responsibilities in educating both staff and physicians in documentation and billing requirements by regulatory agencies and verification that such has taken place.

D. Statement of responsibilities for development and distribution of policies and procedures and methods to be used for charge capture and submission of professional fees that are in compliance with all federal, state, and local laws and regulations.

III. Methods to Ensure Compliance

A. Statement of the mechanism to be used by employees to raise questions and answers and to report possible noncompliance.

B. Methods to achieve appropriate responses and answers to questions regarding compliance and professional billing.

C. The methods to be used to allow confidential reporting of noncompliance.

D. A clear statement that up-coding and unbundling are prohibited.

IV. Sanctions

A list of sanctions of increasing severity that may be invoked against physicians who are found to be in violation of compliance rules and regulations.

# Chapter 9

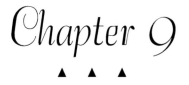

## Mixed Faculty Practice Plan Model in Transition

by Paul H. Rockey, MD, MPH

## Background

Southern Illinois University School of Medicine (SIU-SOM) was founded 25 years ago to help the people of southern Illinois meet their present and future health needs through education, service, and research. As the only "downstate" medical school in Illinois, it serves the teaching and referral medical care needs of a regional population of 2.5 million. Seventy-two first-year medical students are at the parent campus in Carbondale. Their last three years are based 180 miles north in Springfield, Illinois, the state's capital and a medium-sized city of 110,000 with a metropolitan population of a quarter million. (See map on page 68 for location of the main and auxiliary sites for the program.)

SIU-SOM has always emphasized the training of primary care practitioners for the region. It has achieved this goal very successfully and ranks second among all North American medical schools in output of primary care physicians. Since its inception, SIU has graduated 1,364 physicians and trained 917 residents, most of whom have entered careers in primary care.

The school has always had a strong community focus. Initial clinical faculty members were local practitioners and newly recruited full-time faculty were discouraged from clinical practice so as not to compete with them. For the first decade, except for family practice (which was the first fully staffed clinical department), the school recruited only highly specialized practitioners who brought new expertise to the community. However, during the past decade, the school's clinical faculty has expanded significantly and now also includes generalists in internal medicine, pediatrics, and obstetrics/gynecology.

The SIU faculty now totals 136 physician and 33 nonphysician members. There are 260 current residents and fellows. These faculty members see more than 330,000 ambulatory visits per year in 345,000 square feet of clinical space. Annual clinical revenues are approaching $43 million, and the annual clinic expense budget is approximately $21.5 million.

## Organization and Management

The administrative and operational structure of our clinical enterprise is deeply embedded in the academic organization. Paradoxically, individual faculty physicians are free to establish their own fees and work schedules within the constraints of their other faculty duties. All professional service fees must be billed through the school's Medical Services and Research Plan, but individual faculty members enjoy the fruits of their clinical work through a highly individualized contract with the school that pays them a percentage of the dollars they generate.

The organization and management of the faculty practice plan is complex. Some activities are centralized while others are decentralized; some are controlled locally while others are controlled by the parent campus in Carbondale. Direction of major administrative functions is retained within the academic structure. For example, the Dean's Office controls personnel, purchasing, general accounting, bursar, mail, and computing functions and is also responsible for liaison to the University Chancellor, President, and Board of Trustees. The University President's Office controls legal issues (including leases and contracts) and a practice-funded self-insurance program (including risk management services). The University Board of Trustees must approve all leases.

The Office of Clinical Affairs, under an Associate Dean, is responsible for an integrated clinical information system that has common registration, billing, collecting, and accounting systems. Clinical Affairs also manages medical records, medical transcription, the operating and capital budgeting processes, clinical accounting, planning and marketing, space planning, leases, facilities, and managed care contract negotiations. The Associate Dean for Clinical Affairs coordinates interdepartmental activities and hospital relations. Department chairs and their administrators run the outpatient clinics and much of the day-to-day operations at the department or division level using departmental administrative, clinical, and nursing staff.

The Office of Clinical Affairs and department chairs have been responsible for year-to-year, practicewide budgeting and planning. However, individual chairs have a high degree of independence in faculty recruitment.

Governance of the plan is vested with the Dean but is highly influenced by an advisory body: the Medical Service and Research Plan (MSRP) Committee. This committee includes the seven full-time clinical department chairs, the Dean, and six member representatives elected at large.

## Practice Settings

The majority of clinical activities occur in Springfield on the campuses of two independent tertiary hospitals—Memorial Medical Center and Saint John's Hospital. A new 106,000 square foot clinic building on the campus of Memorial Medical Center provides space for general internal medicine, internal medicine subspecialties, general surgery, surgical specialties, obstetrics/gynecology, neurology, dermatology, psychiatry, Alzheimer disease, orthotics, and prosthetics. The other major ambulatory site is in a physician office building (the Pavilion) at St. John's Hospital, where pediatrics, high-risk obstetrics/gynecology, and several medical and surgical subspecialties reside.

## Geographic Location of Elements of SIU-SOM Residency Programs and Rural Clinic Sites

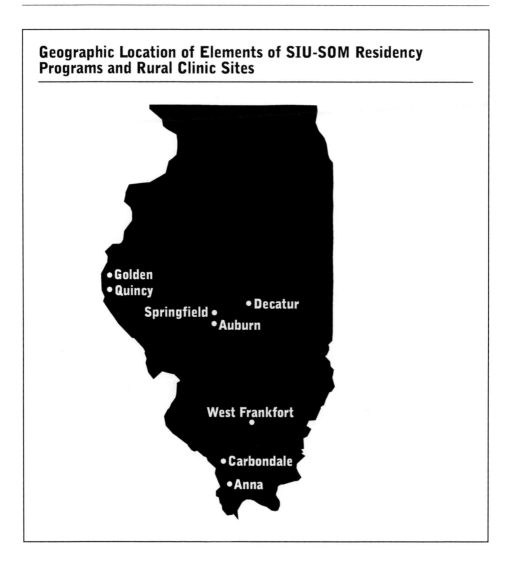

Plastic surgery has space in a privately owned building on the Memorial Medical Center campus. Ophthalmology is in its own facility located between the two hospital campuses and maintains satellites in Jacksonville and Macomb. There is an internal medicine/pediatric clinic 20 miles south of Springfield in Auburn.

The school sponsors four family practice residency programs. The Springfield family practice clinic is housed in a clinic near the Memorial campus. The other three family practice training programs are in the Illinois communities of Quincy, Decatur, and Carbondale. Three of the four programs maintain remote rural clinics.

## Revenue and Expense Distribution

Prior to 1986, the clinical enterprise was integrated into each clinical department's budget. In 1986, major portions of the clinical budget were segregated from departments' activities and organized around a cost-allocation methodology. The cost of clinic personnel, billing and collections, accounting, computing, medical transcription, medical records, space, medical liability, etc. were allocated to each department strictly on the basis of use until 1991. Revenues and expenses were budgeted yearly, establishing an overhead rate prospectively. Every practitioner was subject to this basic overhead rate, and revenues in excess of allocated expenses were credited back to the department in which they were generated. A subsidy from the school was required to balance the budgets of the high expense departments during this period. In 1986, this $2.4 million subsidy accounted for approximately 50 percent of the clinical operating budget. Reduced to $1.7 million in 1992 and to $900,000 in 1996and dwarfed by substantial growth in clinical revenues, it now accounts for less than 5 percent of the clinical budget.

In 1992, allocation methodologies were modified. While the overhead recovery, in total, was adequate to pay all expenses, it was maldistributed, because it accumulated at the department level. Thus, departments with lower expenses (primarily surgical) had surplus funds while high-expense departments (e.g., primary care) operated at deficits. We changed the allocation formulas to distribute expenses for computing, telecommunications, accounting, and some billing functions as a percentage of receipts. This strategy was expanded in 1994, when we adopted a "global budget" that pooled all additional revenues to fund only the highest priority incremental expenses.

## Faculty Compensation

Faculty compensation has two components: academic base salary and clinical income. The academic base is established using Association of American Medical Colleges guidelines and is reduced to recognize release time to practice. Clinical income is based on a percentage of fees generated. For faculty members who are predominantly clinical, an additional overhead assessment may fund their academic base. There are no clinical practice "guarantees" except during the initial 6-12 months of practice, when a new member may draw advances on his or her future clinical income from a revolving fund. A graduated ceiling on salary has been in place for many years. This has not worked well and is now largely circumvented by establishing unrealistically high ceilings.

Our compensation plan and allocation methodologies have both strengths and weaknesses and have resulted in both successes and failures.

### Successes and Strengths

▲ Because increased clinical productivity results directly in increased compensation, the most salient success of our organization is our highly productive clinical faculty. Based on data from a 1992 AAMC survey, SIU faculty are two to three times as clinically productive as the average clinical faculty.

▲ Attending physician availability and resultant opportunities for student and resident mentoring in the hospital and clinics is greatly enhanced.

▲ We have no debt in the faculty practice plan and, because the system operates entirely on a cash basis, there is no risk related to paying faculty practice income.

▲ The clinical information system is entirely integrated, with common registration, billing and accounting, chart tracking, and other functions. This sophisticated, though not state-of-the-art, system has eliminated redundant multiple systems and has allowed for an integrated budgeting process.

▲ The faculty practice plan has been able to direct a significant portion of its budget to support the school. About 10 percent of clinical revenue is distributed equally to the Dean and the departments to support academic programs, and an additional 5 percent is gleaned by most divisions for similar purposes.

▲ Despite the lack of centralized authority, the practice has achieved nearly universal participation in several managed care programs. This is probably because most faculty members recognize their financial interdependency and because strong internal referral patterns exist.

### Failures and Weaknesses

▲ Tying faculty compensation directly to clinical earnings may encourage and reward clinical activity at the expense of more formal academic pursuits, such as research.

▲ A production-oriented ("do more, make more") compensation structure will create perverse incentives as our managed care activity increases.

▲ Our compensation scheme and flow of funds, by rewarding individual achievement, has not fostered group behavior.

▲ We lack "single pen" authority for executing managed care contracts, thus diluting our negotiating position.

▲ We have diffuse responsibility and authority for managing the clinical enterprise, with some authority in the President's office, some in the Dean's office, some in the departmental structure, and some in the Office of Clinical Affairs.

▲ There are significant inefficiencies in the clinical enterprise related to department and division staffing and the lack of shared staff.

▲ We have not accumulated any savings, reserves, or contingency funds because of our month-to-month cash accounting system.

▲ Revenue estimates have to be very accurate to prevent shortfalls, because the overhead rate (charged to clinical income) is set prospectively from year to year.

▲ Personnel policies of the university and the State of Illinois civil service system are not necessarily supportive or responsive to our clinical endeavors. Furthermore, these personnel policies may limit compensation for individuals critical to the success of the organization and operation of the clinic.

▲ We lack an ability to create incentives for performance in areas, such as customer service, medical transcription, and collections, where this would be beneficial.

▲ State and university rules and regulations are oftentimes slow and cumbersome and make simple administrative tasks much more complex than those found in the private sector.

▲ We lack a strong public perception of our clinical capabilities because of the lack of a group practice identity.

▲ Because of all these factors, our 160 clinicians do not enjoy the "clout" that a multispecialty group practice of our size should enjoy in our region.

## Changes Implemented

Significant progress has been achieved toward group processes and behavior over the past five or six years. With the recruitment of an Associate Dean for Clinical Affairs in 1991, the Clinical Chairs Committee was established. The department and central plan administrators have also met regularly during the same period. An environment of collaborative planning and problem solving has been created.

In 1992 and 1993, we made a significant push toward the creation of a shared clinical identity by adopting the name "SIU Physicians & Surgeons." An image awareness campaign, targeted to the general population and to referring physicians, highlighted our clinical practice of medicine and surgery as well as our mission to teach the next generation of physicians.

## Changes Anticipated

By 1994, MSRP, School of Medicine, and department leadership knew that change was imperative if we were to maintain our market presence and educational mission in an increasingly competitive environment. Seven subcommittees were convened to address issues of governance; faculty compensation/tenure/promotion; managed care; finance; personnel; management practices, and external affairs. Among the recommendations made by these subcommittees were:

▲ The clinical enterprise should have a greater degree of self-governance.

▲ The governance structure should be accountable to the membership of the practice plan.

▲ Market-driven, productivity-based compensation should be maintained.

▲ An adequate primary care base should be developed.

▲ Systems should be developed to ensure success in the managed care arena.

▲ Opportunities for cost efficiency should be maximized.

▲ Reserves to fund group strategic initiatives should be established.

▲ The personnel system should be responsive to the needs of a clinical practice.

Among the seven subcommittees, there was general recognition that our current, individual-practitioner model was rapidly becoming obsolete. In order to ensure future success, we had to move from a model that offered short-term, personal financial gain to one that provided for long-term group stability. Thus, one theme consistently emerged: The physicians must become a group practice.

Late in the summer of 1994, the Committee for Restructuring the Faculty Practice Plan was formed and identified several objectives that a group practice should achieve:

▲ Increase our negotiating leverage and access to managed care contracts.

▲ Create reserves to fund strategic initiatives.

▲ Streamline shared administrative, financial, and operating systems.

▲ Improve access and convenience for our patients.

▲ Increase our security through group affiliation.

▲ Develop a compensation model that furthers our group goals while continuing to reward individual productivity.

The Restructuring Committee also identified a number of corollaries to these objectives. First, our clinical practice expenses and revenues must be separated from our other activities (e.g., academic missions). Without this separation, we cannot accurately account for and manage clinical expenses. Second, the good of the group must supersede the good of the individual. Third, management responsibility must be delegated to a small group that can act on behalf of our membership, yet be accountable to us all. Fourth, we must maintain a broad patient base for our teaching programs. Finally, in the eyes of all our "customers," we must look and act like a group.

The Restructuring Committee has identified five key arenas for development:

▲ Legal structure

▲ Governance and representation

▲ Flow of funds

▲ Management services

▲ Integration of clinical practice and academic programs

### Legal Structure
Several alternative legal structures were considered and debated, ranging from full employment by the school to complete disassociation and establishment of a professional corporation. The model selected is a not-for-profit, university-related organization. This type of organization will afford greater administrative authority and self-governance than our current structure, while allowing us to maintain some of the significant advantages we enjoy today. We have obtained university and school approval for this new entity to be incorporated as "SIU Physicians & Surgeons." the Articles of Incorporation have been filed with the Secretary of State, and we are preparing a request for an IRS letter ruling to support the group's not-for-profit status

## Governance

The Restructuring Committee agreed that a governance that is more representative of the clinical faculty and that could move with unity and speed is imperative. The committee proposed an 11-member, constituency-elected board of trustees, replacing the current MSRP Committee. Representation is as follows:

▲ One primary care representative (general internal medicine, family medicine, general pediatrics, and general obstetrics)

▲ One medical specialty representative (internal medicine, neurology, psychiatry, and pediatric subspecialties)

▲ One surgical specialty representative (surgery, obstetrics/gynecology)

▲ One at-large representative

▲ The Dean

▲ Three clinical chairs

▲ Three outside directors

In addition to the board, specific-purpose committees will be established to cover such areas as finance, managed care, faculty compensation, quality assurance, and so forth. Although chaired by a member of the board, the committees would be composed of other plan members, thus expanding faculty input into the management of the clinical enterprise.

Responsibilities of the board and the committee structure will include overall practice management, strategic planning, resource/revenue allocation, managed care contracting, and establishment of practicewide policy. Adoption of the new governance structure is independent of adopting a new legal structure and will likely precede it.

## Flow of Funds

The Restructuring Committee is just beginning to consider the flow of funds. The fundamental question is: Who owns clinical revenue? Currently, revenues belong to individuals. In the proposed model, revenues, after all expenses are paid, will belong to the group, with strong incentives for individual productivity. Clinical operating expenses would be covered first. Any excess will be distributed to group practice reserves, department/division funds, and clinical compensation. In addition to an academic base salary, each practitioner's clinical compensation will have two components: clinical base salary and clinical incentive. The details of this program are being developed.

## Uncharted Territories

The last two critical issues facing the practice plan are management structure and integration with the academic program.

In summary, the current Medical Services and Research Plan is a liability in our increasingly competitive environment. Group direction, economies of scale, rapid decision making, and faculty involvement are crucial to future success. Although many questions remain unanswered, we have developed a governance structure that will enable us to achieve the benefits of group practice without losing the incentives for productivity that have made us strong.

*Paul H. Rockey, MD, MPH, is Associate Dean for Clinical Affairs, School of Medicine, Southern Illinois University, Springfield.*

# Chapter 10

▲ ▲ ▲

## Practice Plan Associates:
## A Plan in Transition

by Joel A. Kaplan, MD, and Milton H. Sisselman, MS

### Organization and Management

Although Mount Sinai School of Medicine matriculated its first group of medical students in September 1968, its initial faculty practice plan was not established until July 1973. During this transition period the on-campus clinical faculty consisted of a small full-time cadre (with fixed compensation levels) and a larger group of geographic full-time members with no restraints on practice earnings.

During the period described here, full-time meant a physician faculty member who devoted his or her full professional effort (academic and clinical) to the Mount Sinai Institutions for a fixed annual compensation. Compensation level was based on a salary guide adopted by the Mount Sinai Board of Trustees and was related to academic rank. From time to time, the salary guide was upgraded by the Board. Salary supplements were not permitted. Any private practice income generated by the full-time physician, less overhead charges, was deposited in a department fund used for education, research, and other approved purposes. In some institutions, this faculty category is defined as "strict full-time."

Geographic full-time (GFT) referred to a physician who received a part-time annual salary from the Mount Sinai Institutions and who committed at least 75 percent of his or her time to professional activities within the medical school and/or hospital. In addition, a GFT physician could engage in private practice, in on-campus facilities (for which an overhead charge was assessed), with minimal restrictions on the amount of practice income the physician might retain.

Early attempts at forming a faculty practice plan, with restrictions on compensation and other limitations, were appealed to the Board of Trustees by the geographic full-time faculty, which effectively stopped the process. With the passage of time and the growing need to increase and strengthen the full-time clinical staff (to accommodate a larger student body), the Board of Trustees accepted the recommendation of the Dean to implement a plan agreeable to most constituencies effective July 1, 1973. This plan was designated as the Medical Service Plan (MSP). In effect, the geographic full-time faculty group was to be phased out.

Its members were given an opportunity to convert to full-time status or move off campus and become members of the voluntary faculty and staff.

In 1976, under the auspices of a Board of Trustees special committee, the School of Medicine undertook a major institutionwide self-study effort that included the Medical Service Plan. As a result of recommendations made by this committee and approved by the Board, the Medical Service Plan was revised and modifications were introduced as of July 1, 1976. Underlying the recommendations was the general consensus that the original MSP needed change to:

▲ Attract more physicians to full-time work.

▲ Retain more physicians in full-time status after they built up their practices.

▲ Divert some portion of practice income to support basic science departments and general educational facilities.

As originally established, the practice plan governance structure dealt largely with internal issues pertaining to the operation of the plan. While subject to a set of School of Medicine-approved rules and procedures (relating to income flow and distribution) and applicable to all participants, in the main each group or individual practitioner functioned in a discrete manner unrelated to other groups or individuals (department-based plan).

Recognizing that changes taking place in the health care arena required an organizational arrangement that would permit FPA—the plan name was changed to Faculty Practice Associates in May 1984—to respond to new initiatives in a prompt and more unified manner, FPA participants, in June 1986 adopted a new set of governance by-laws. The by-laws were subsequently approved by the President of the Medical Center and were made effective as of July 1,1986.

An FPA Administrative Office under the direction of an Executive Director/Vice President for Faculty Practice provides staff support to the President of FPA and to FPA governing bodies. This office also coordinates implementation of FPA policies and procedures, monitors use of assigned practice space, oversees and supports billing and collection activities of the various FPA practices, and performs other administrative functions (federated plan).

At the practice or department level, FPA is decentralized. Under general guidelines established by the FPA governing bodies, each clinical department is responsible for administration and operation of assigned practice areas, including billing and collection activities. Practice receipts are deposited into discrete accounts listed in the name of the FPA participant or group and are maintained in the Financial Division of the School of Medicine. Disbursements from these accounts are made in accordance with established guidelines governing participation in FPA.

## Governance

Governance of the FPA is now vested in a President, a Vice President, an FPA Executive Council, and an FPA Assembly.

### FPA Executive Council

The Executive Council consists of 11 members, including the President and the Vice President. No clinical department may have more than one representative on the FPA Executive Council (including the President and the Vice President). After the President and the Vice President are elected (following a procedure defined in the FPA By-laws of Governance), nine additional members of the FPA Executive Council are selected from three categories:

▲ Category A—Four members chosen from the four departments with the highest gross receipts.

▲ Category B—Two members chosen from the two departments with the largest number of participants (unless chosen for Category A).

▲ Category C—Three members chosen from a list of departments (selected in random order) not otherwise represented on the FPA Executive Council.

The President and the Vice President serve on the FPA Executive Council for four years. Category A, B, and C members serve for two years. The President chairs the FPA Executive Council, which meets monthly.

### FPA Assembly

All clinical departments are represented on the FPA Assembly. The size of a department's delegation is based on its number of FPA participants as of June of each year.

| Number of FPA Participants in Department | Number of Representatives in FPA Assembly |
|---|---|
| 1-9 | 1 |
| 10-24 | 2 |
| 25 or more | 3 |

In each department, the chair or his or her designee is an appointed member. Departments eligible for two or three members elect additional representatives from their FPA participants. The Vice President of FPA chairs the FPA Assembly, which meets quarterly.

## Practice Settings

When FPA was first organized some 20 years ago, practice activities were conducted in various department- or hospital-owned facilities. Although it had been a declared part of institutional policy to encourage expansion of FPA practices, accommodating new FPA participants and the concomitant increased patient population put a severe strain on existing facilities. This reached a critical point in 1984. With the strong recommendation of the President of the Medical Center, the Board of Trustees authorized conversion of an existing 16-story, on-campus building that would, upon completion, allow for consolidation of all FPA practices into a single facility. In addition to providing expanded quarters, it was felt that this building would:

▲ Provide FPA with a specific physical identity.

▲ Enhance referrals among FPA participants.

▲ Project a more positive image of FPA as an organized faculty group practice.

The first phase of construction was completed in November 1987 with occupancy of four floors. Since that time, FPA practices have expanded onto additional floors on a scheduled basis, and, by the end of 1997, it is planned that more than 55 FPA practices will be housed on 13 floors of this dedicated facility.

Although it was intended that most practices would be located in the FPA building, certain practices (namely, radiology, radiation/oncology, and rehabilitation medicine), because of their special physical requirements, could not be accommodated and are housed in hospital space. Appropriate reimbursement is made to the hospital for FPA practice-related services. Also, a number of primary care units are located in off-campus sites.

To help meet FPA's contribution toward the debt service of the bonds issued to help finance the building's renovation costs, the FPA governing bodies authorized an annual assessment of 5 percent of all FPA practice gross receipts for this purpose. This was in addition to other overhead assessments, as noted below.

## Revenue and Expense Distribution

Ambulatory practice activities of FPA participants are conducted primarily in offices located in the FPA building dedicated for this purpose. As hospital attending physicians, FPA members may also admit patients to the hospital or be called in as consultants.

All full-time members of the faculty, upon recommendation of their department chair, are eligible to participate in FPA. FPA participants may operate on an individual or group basis. If they function as a group, there is usually agreement in advance on how available salary supplements and other FPA benefits are to be distributed. All patient care-related receipts generated by FPA participants are deposited into a separate account established for each individual or group participating in the plan.

A fixed percentage of gross receipts is deducted and allocated to the School Equalization Fund (Dean's Fund). This fund may be used at the discretion of the Dean in support of School of Medicine activities. With the concurrence of FPA, the Dean has specified his intention to use these dollars to support the basic science departments, the library, and related academic activities that are of general benefit to the entire School of Medicine community.

A direct overhead charge covering expenses required by a participant to generate practice income plus a fixed percentage for indirect costs are also deducted.

The amount remaining is designated as "adjusted gross income." Under the plan, subject to the approval of the department chair, various charges or disbursements may be made against the adjusted gross income, for example:

▲ A percentage of base salary and related fringe benefits.

▲ An expense allowance.

▲ Premium cost of added disability insurance.

▲ Access to a fixed percentage of adjusted gross income (up to 10 percent).

▲ These items are all subject to income tax and are included on annual W-2 forms.

The amount remaining after deducting the allowable charges from the adjusted gross income is designated as the "residual balance." Half of the residual balance is allocated to a department fund. In consultation with plan participants, the department chair may authorize expenditures from these funds in accordance with institutional policy.

The remaining 50 percent is available for supplementation of the participant's base salary. This supplement is negotiated on an annual basis between the participant and the department chair and is subject to the approval of the Dean.

## Faculty Compensation

As full-time members of the faculty, FPA participants receive a base salary, listed in the salary range appropriate for each academic rank as approved by the Board of Trustees, on which institutional fringe benefits are paid or calculated. Base salaries may be derived from various sources available to department chairs (including practice income) and are usually adjusted on an annual basis.

Under existing policies, FPA participants may supplement their incomes on an annual basis up to a maximum of 100 percent of base salary. In addition, under special criteria approved by the Compensation Committee of the Board of Trustees, qualified FPA participants may exceed the 100 percent limit through a year-end adjustment.

## General Comments

As we endeavor to respond to environmental initiatives, now in place or in the planning stage, designed to constrain medical care costs and modify our health care delivery system, it becomes evident that FPA, as an ongoing entity, will have to consider various policy and operational changes if we are to survive and prosper.

### Policy Issues

▲ Modify governance to strengthen decision-making processes, improve response time to managed care organizations, and enhance relationships with voluntary and alliance physicians.

▲ Restructure FPA to accommodate alternative forms of payment. (capitation, global contracts, etc.)

▲ Plan how to accommodate potential reduction in practice income.

▲ Arrange to share income among practices to more equitably balance participation in FPA.

▲ Balance growth between a need for a larger primary care base and development of specialty services.

▲ Decide what effort or resources, if any, FPA should devote to the development of satellites or other outreach programs.

▲ Develop an ambulatory care quality assurance programming base on continuous quality improvement principles.

▲ Begin clinical outcomes research programs.

### Operational Issues

▲ Develop a more uniform financial reporting and management information system that reflects activity of practices and accommodates future reimbursement changes in the future.

▲ Improve arrangements to share facilities, personnel, and other resources among different practices to reduce costs and enhance efficiency.

▲ Incorporate off-site physicians into a "practice without walls" arrangement or add additional practice space.

▲ Incorporate hospital outpatient facilities into the FPA structure.

▲ Coordinate activities with Mount Sinai Hospital, Mount Sinai Health System, and Management Service Organization to establish an integrated health care delivery system in the next five years.

## Epilogue

The growing influence of managed care and capitation payments on the delivery of health care services moved the FPA leadership, in June 1995, to appoint a special Ad Hoc Committee to consider how best FPA might respond to these compelling issues.

In reviewing the current governance arrangement, it became evident that, above all, the FPA decision-making process had to be improved. The need to respond promptly, and for the group as a whole, to managed care and related initiatives was obvious, as HMOs, PPOs, and other managed care companies continue to increase their share of the medical care marketplace.

The Ad Hoc Committee recognized early on that the burden of this responsibility rested with the department chairs. Thus, it became evident that the chairs must constitute the key component of the proposed new governance body—the Board of Governors.

The proposed plan does not allow for "surrogates" to represent a chair. Because all board decisions regarding managed care arrangements will be binding on all FPA members, attendance at board meetings is in the best interests of each chair. The assumption is that the chairs must "buy in" on board decisions and assist and cooperate in their implementation. Only through full and personal involvement in board deliberations and voting on actions taken can this be accomplished.

Other amendments to existing rules are also being offered, but the expanded role of the chairs in FPA decision making is the signal modification being put forward.

The recommendations of the Ad Hoc Committee are under review by various FPA and other institutional groups and should be resolved by the middle of 1997.

*Joel A. Kaplan, MD, is Senior Vice President, Clinical Affairs; Chairman and Horace W. Goldsmith Professor, Department of Anesthesiology; and President, Faculty Practice Associates; Mount Sinai Medical Center, New York, New York. Milton H. Sisselman, MS, serves as an Executive Consultant to Faculty Practice Associates.*

# Chapter 11

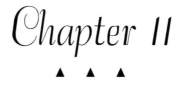

## Centralization Key Goal of Faculty Practice Plan

by Rein Saral, MD, and Garland D. Perdue, MD

### Introduction and History

Fifty years ago, Emory University School of Medicine relied heavily on a small number of salaried faculty in its clinical departments, augmented by full-time physicians located on or near the Emory campus and in Emory University Hospital. The latter faculty members received no salary and supported themselves by remuneration for clinical services rendered to private patients. Salaried faculty members supplemented their incomes by a more limited private practice. All private practice revenues were the property of individual physicians. The faculty was further enlarged by a large number of volunteer members, whose contributions varied from significant commitment to occasional limited activity.

A long-range planning committee appointed by the President of the University reported in 1946. Implementation of three important recommendations of that committee has had a major impact on further development of Emory University School of Medicine:

▲ Concentration of basic science and much clinical teaching activity on the Emory campus from previously scattered locations.

▲ Development of research activities in laboratory facilities to be constructed on the Emory campus.

▲ Creation of a plan providing practice opportunities for faculty members and financial contributions to the School of Medicine.

The faculty organization was created on January 1,1953, as the Emory University Clinic, a general partnership of a small number of both salaried and full-time physicians, including the chairs of the departments of medicine and surgery. Antecedent individuals and groups of internists, surgeons, surgical oncologists, orthopedists, and thoracic surgeons were represented in the 17 founding partners. Other faculty subsequently joined in the formative period, but several important departments were not represented for several years. The Emory University Clinic eventually included all faculty providing services for remuneration by patients and third-party payers. A second practice plan was subsequently created to receive third-party payments in public institutions so as to avoid commingling public and private funds. Membership in this group largely, but not completely, overlapped that of the Emory University Clinic.

## Evolution

Several important principles were established in the formative period:

▲ The group would be self-governing as an autonomous legal entity. Emory University repeatedly disclaimed an interest in direct involvement in the provision of medical services. This eventually led to shortening the name to the Emory Clinic.

▲ All private practice by members of the faculty would be under the auspices of the Emory Clinic.

▲ Faculty appointment would be prerequisite to membership in the Clinic.

▲ Financial contributions to the School of Medicine and the University would be defined by contract. It would be in the mutual interest of the Clinic and the University for this to be a multiyear contract.

▲ From the beginning, the Emory Clinic was defined as a multispecialty group practice, with centralized business administration, medical records, and billing and collection functions.

▲ The internal organization would be with sections that correspond to established academic departments. Clinic policies and procedures would supersede those of individual sections, but sections generally would have great autonomy in clinical assignments, internal scheduling, determination of personnel needs, and distribution of internal surplus earnings.

▲ Revenues would be retained by the sections, which would be expected to pay their operating costs as well as their share of allocated costs for University and School of Medicine payments and for the costs of centralized administration.

▲ Physician compensation would be based largely on productivity, as modified by seniority and faculty rank, contributions to scholarship, and uncompensated service to the University.

These principles are not inviolate, but close adherence has been maintained through the evolution of the Emory Clinic to the present.

## Present Status of the Emory Clinic

The Emory Clinic has grown consistently in numbers, size of facilities, individual productivity, annual revenues, and monetary support to the School of Medicine. It is presently comprises approximately 800 physicians and 2,000 employees, including physicians' assistants, nurse practitioners, nurse clinicians, and technicians in various disciplines. Facilities include approximately 600,000 square feet in buildings on the Emory campus, approximately 168,000 square feet in multiple facilities at a branch location at Crawford Long Hospital in downtown Atlanta, and growing satellites in neighborhoods and suburbs. The latter are in leased space. A full range of ambulatory services, including ambulatory surgery, radiation oncology, and clinical laboratory facilities, is provided.

## Legal Structure

The original Emory University Clinic became the Emory Clinic when the word "University" was dropped from the name to emphasize the legal autonomy of the organization. It was for many years a general partnership. Change to a professional corporation was considered and rejected, but conversion to a not-for-profit, tax-exempt corporation was initiated in 1992, with merger of the assets and accounts receivable of the partnership in 1993 and the first year of operation as the new entity in 1994.

## Governance

The original partnership agreement specified central governance in an administrative committee. Section heads were *ex officio* members, and other members were appointed to give weighted representation to larger sections. Department chairs were not required to be section heads, and some appointed deputies to serve in this capacity. In actual practice, evolution achieved the present practice of all department chairs serving as titular and functional section heads.

## Committees

A number of standing medical staff committees exist, and the advice and recommendations of these committees are sought and carefully considered as to policies, procedures, rules, and regulations of the clinic.

The Administrative Committee, as previously constituted, acted on the recommendations of the clinic director and the standing committees, and these actions required approval of the partners. The ideal of the Greek word *polis* became increasingly difficult to achieve with increasing size of the group, however, and, in practice, the decisions of the administrative committee were rarely contested. The partners recognized this by ceding governing authority to a successor Executive Committee, with section heads (department chairs) holding seats *ex officio* and twelve members elected as at-large representatives serving three-year terms. The Dean of the School of Medicine serves *ex officio* without vote. When the Emory Clinic became a tax-exempt corporation, the composition of this committee remained the same, but it is now designated the Board of Directors. In effect, the Board of Directors is the decision-making body. Former partners are now designated senior members, and new senior members are ratified by vote. At-large members of the Board are elected by vote.

The Clinic Director is selected by the Executive Vice President of the Woodruff Health Sciences Center from a short list of nominees provided by an executive committee of the Board of Directors, acting as a search committee, and this nomination is ratified by vote. In all other matters, decisions are made by the Board of Directors of the Corporation.

After four years of service, members are eligible for election as senior members upon nomination by their sections and approval by the Board of Directors. Associate professors may be nominated after two years, and professors after one year. New senior members may be admitted upon recommendation of the Board of Directors and by affirmative vote of 80 percent of members eligible to vote, provided that not more than 10 percent of the members eligible to vote cast votes against the proposed senior members. Only senior members may vote.

## Management

Management of the clinic is by an administrative/management staff. The chief executive officer is the Clinic Director, who is required to be a physician. The Clinic Director may select associate directors, and the Executive Administrator and his or her management staff are accountable to the physician leadership.

## Practice Patterns

Historically, membership has comprised the specialists of the faculty, and patients were preselected and referred by other physicians. Acceptance of self-referred patients was gradually permitted over the past decade, but most services were heavily concentrated in tertiary and quaternary care. As managed care has assumed growing prominence, it has become increasingly clear that choice of physician and specialist may be limited by terms of a managed care contract. Several important decisions were made in the past five years:

▲ Primary care physicians would be incorporated into a new department of family practice and in departments of medicine, pediatrics, and obstetrics/gynecology.

▲ These physicians would be "distributed," along with specialists as needed, in branch clinics having a hub-and-spoke configuration (see figure below). The "hubs" consist of large multispecialty clinics. The "spokes" refer to smaller primary care physician practice sites that surround the larger clinics.

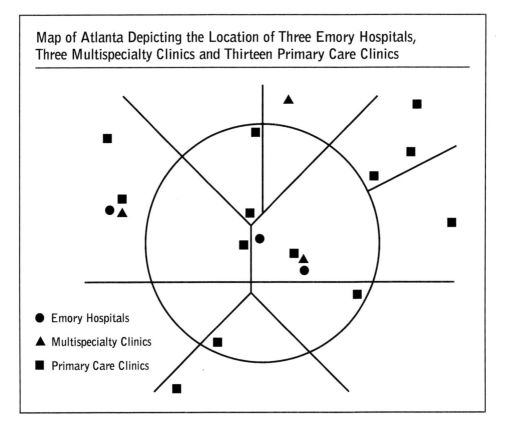

**Map of Atlanta Depicting the Location of Three Emory Hospitals, Three Multispecialty Clinics and Thirteen Primary Care Clinics**

● Emory Hospitals

▲ Multispecialty Clinics

■ Primary Care Clinics

▲ A systemwide electronic network would be established to distribute clinical information from a clinical data repository. Eventual integration of clinical, financial, administrative, and outcomes data is planned.

▲ The organization, jointly with the two Emory-owned hospitals, would initiate marketing activities and would compete vigorously for contracts to provide services under the provisions of managed care plans as desired by large employers and/or administered by third-party payers.

▲ Renewed attention to cost efficiency would be achieved through business "reengineering" and total quality management.

▲ Capital required for construction of new enlarged facilities on the Emory University campus would be diverted to these new programs.

▲ Financial reporting systems would be enhanced to address the anticipated growth in managed care contracting, and the accounting method changed from cash to accrual.

## Academic Responsibilities

The clinic founders recognized that individuals were unlikely to be able to contribute in equal measure to scholarship and research, teaching, and clinical services. Balance would be best achieved at the division or the department level, with individuals contributing in accordance with preferences, talents, and availability. Clinic membership has included those who are considered "full-time" in clinical service and scholarship and those who are "part-time." The former are expected to provide no less than 20 percent of their time and efforts to teaching, research, or contribution to scholarship. In actual practice, this has averaged about one-third time and effort, but these members are available on a daily basis for clinical services and continuity of care to patients. "Part-time" members, on the other hand, spend the majority of their time and effort in research, scholarly effort, and teaching in the clinical services at Grady Memorial Hospital or the Atlanta VA Medical Center, both major teaching affiliates in the integrated teaching program. Part-time members receive a base salary from the School of Medicine or from another institution. Consequently, the number of full-time equivalent physicians is approximately one-half the total number.

## Revenue and Expense Distribution

Revenues received by the Emory Clinic are assigned to the sections generating the services and to individuals when payments are designated. Undesignated payments, including capitation revenues, are assigned by an equity allocation relating the services provided to an approved clinic fee schedule. The flow of funds then follows a general model:

▲ Payments to the university for a building fund and for the school of medicine are a contractual obligation based on a percentage of revenues. A mild progressive tax system is used in which a formula specifies that more prosperous individuals and sections pay more than 100 percent of their obligation and less prosperous individuals and sections pay less than their obligation. The percentages are recommended by the Clinic Director, reviewed by the Finance Committee, and approved by the Board of Directors annually.

▲ Central administrative costs are determined as a percentage of revenues, and each section pays this percentage of its revenues as its share of these costs. More prosperous sections thus pay more of the costs—in effect, a progressive tax.

▲ The direct operating expenses of the section, including supplies, salaries of employed personnel, and physician base salaries, are paid.

▲ Certain shared services are allocated to the sections in proportion to use. Examples include building maintenance and utilities (based on square footage) and telephone and electronic network (based on direct charges plus a share reflecting the number of user outlets).

▲ After all obligations are met, it is anticipated a surplus will remain. For most of its history, the Emory Clinic used the cash basis for accounting. All surplus funds were distributed under a formula that provided a general clinic share of a designated amount, the remainder being distributed within the sections. This system is being modified to permit some retention of capital by the clinic. Sections may also retain capital for equipment needs and for a contribution to department funds.

It is important to stress that all financial systems and formulas are reviewed and modified, if necessary, annually to try to maintain fairness in the face of constantly changing circumstances.

### Faculty Compensation

Our goal is to recruit *and retain* desired faculty members. To this end, compensation is market-based initially and largely productivity-based in subsequent years. Faculty rank and seniority; contributions to scholarship through teaching, research, and publications; and service to the clinic are given weight as well, and compensation varies from one section to another to maintain peer comparability in the same discipline. Generally, we achieve compensation for faculty that places them in the upper quartile of faculty members elsewhere.

## Discussion

The authors have a combined 12 years' experience in executive leadership of the Emory Clinic. We have confidence in this model and believe it is flexible enough to adapt to a changing environment. Strategic planning is an essential part of executive responsibility, and changes are likely to occur in several areas.

Legal structure and governance are considered optimum at present. While the majority of the Board of Directors comprises *ex officio* section heads (department chairs), faculty interests are represented and balance is maintained by election of at-large representatives to the Board. These members serve three years and may be reelected. Concerns about the possibility of cabalistic governance have not been realized. Faculty member input is also achieved by the large number of standing committees appointed by the Clinic Director from faculty members in clinical departments. These committees consider issues and refinements of policies and procedures, and their recommendations are given great weight by the Board of Directors.

Management by an administrative staff and centralized operations are also considered to be optimum and essential to the efficient performance of a multispecialty clinic.

Centrifugal forces arising from department concerns exist, but no serious effort to have these become overriding issues has arisen. It is anticipated that, within the framework of general policies and procedures, sections (departments) will continue to have significant autonomy. More development of interdepartmental centers for clinical efficiency may actually diminish department territoriality.

Incorporation of primary care physicians and the requirements of clinical efficiency in a managed care environment create a set of interrelated issues. Payment mechanisms incorporating global capitation and payment as a percentage of premium for a defined population add to these issues. We believe the issues can be addressed, bearing in mind historical principles outlined earlier in this chapter. Indeed, we believe the historical development of a corporate culture *must* be taken into account as changes are initiated and that change should be as leisurely and evolutionary as external requirements permit.

Clearly, some physicians are being added whose contributions to the school of medicine and the clinic will be clinical service, with limited or minimal requirements for contributions to scholarship and research. As pointed out earlier, we have accommodated service weighted toward clinical activity, but with expectation of some contribution to teaching and scholarship. Some relaxation of this expectation will have to be accepted, pending redefinition of teaching in the ambulatory setting and of the place of "role models" as exemplars of good medical practice. Further, the school of medicine may well consider categories of faculty and criteria for promotion beyond those of the tracks (research, clinical, and tenure) presently in use. We believe it desirable to minimize perception of multiple classes of faculty, because all contribute to the needs of the school of medicine.

Expense allocations for the university, the school of medicine, and central administration are subject to annual revision, and future revisions may well require forgiveness of some portion of these obligations to accommodate start-up costs of primary care practices and satellite clinics. Operating losses may also have to be accommodated until these operations reach break-even status as freestanding entities. The present progressive tax system can probably be revised to meet these needs.

Financial productivity has been heavily weighted in determination of physician compensation in the past as a reflection of the fee-for-service environment. This has been required to maintain relative comparability to competitive opportunities in the Atlanta and other marketplaces. Line-of-service capitation agreements can be allocated by the equity of the providers of the services rendered, but, as more global capitation or percentage-of-premium agreements are reached, increasing weight will have to be given to efficiency of practice and appropriate utilization of resources. Seniority, faculty rank, and contributions to teaching and scholarship will continue to carry weight, subject to the accommodation required for new faculty and primary care activities in satellite locations. The net effect will likely be a decrease in compensation to previously highly rewarded specialists, but, as this is expected to be a widespread phenomenon, it is probable that comparability can be maintained as the marketplace evolves. Finally, capital requirements are likely to continue to increase for such needs as telecommunication and electronic information services. Preservation of capital, rather than distribution of earnings, will require more attention than has been traditional. Our financial systems will accommodate this revision.

Controversy in the midst of change is inevitable, but we believe it can be resolved with the well-formulated principles that have served us well through 40 years of continuous growth and development.

*Rein Saral, MD, is Clinic Director and CEO, Emory Clinic, Inc., Atlanta, Georgia. Garland D. Perdue, MD, is former Clinic Director.*

# Chapter 12

▲ ▲ ▲

## Pediatrics Faculty Practice Plan
## Looks to Managed Care Future

by James A. Menke, MD, Richard E. McClead, MD,
and Mitchell Wheller, BS, MHA

## Introduction

Children's Hospital in Columbus, Ohio, incorporated in 1892. In 1916, it affiliated with the Ohio State University-College of Medicine (OSU-COM). The pediatric academic program did not grow, however, until pediatrics, a division of the internal medicine department, received department status in 1941.[1] Since then, the Department of Pediatrics at OSU-COM has been based at the Children's Hospital.

Over the years, the pediatric faculty consisted mainly of pediatricians in private practice. In exchange for their teaching efforts, these faculty members received a small stipend and a clinical faculty appointment from OSU-COM. Eventually, a few full-time pediatric faculty members were hired. Their offices were in Children's Hospital. They received a small salary and a regular faculty appointment at OSU-COM. These faculty members supplemented their income with patient care dollars. They billed and collected patient care revenues for their own use. While scholarly activity was encouraged, the primary focus of these faculty members was the private practice of medicine.

A few faculty members, especially procedure-oriented subspecialists, developed large private practices and significant personal incomes. This limited the ability of the department to recruit new faculty. It also led to misallocation of effort. Incentives favored patient care activity, with little emphasis on teaching and research. It also created a two-class system of health care. "Paying" patients were seen in private faculty offices. "Clinic" or "service" patients (i.e., poor people) were seen in hospital clinics by the pediatric housestaff supervised by the faculty.

In 1978, a new chair of the department of pediatrics was hired. He was charged with developing the academic program, including research. To accomplish this goal, the new chair recognized the need to control patient care revenues and the allocation of faculty effort between patient care, teaching, and research. To that end, he established a committee to conduct a feasibility study. The committee's purpose was to develop a unified academic department practice plan. In 1981, after a year study, the practice plan of the department of pediatrics was incorporated. This planning period was important, because a unified practice plan for the department of pediatrics was a new and threatening concept. The plan is known as the Pediatric Academic Association, Inc. (PAA).

All faculty members were given the opportunity to join PAA. Faculty members who were in private practice were offered a three-year salary guarantee as an incentive to join. Initially, all faculty members, except for a neonatologist, an endocrinologist, an infectious disease specialist, and the four-person section of pediatric cardiology, joined PAA. Within three years, the section of pediatric cardiology joined. The other individuals have not. Since 1981, all new pediatric faculty members must join PAA. The start-up costs for PAA were secured by a no interest, five-year loan from Children's Hospital for $500,000. (Today, this loan agreement would not be permitted under the federal safe harbor laws.) PAA was the first department practice plan at OSU. Today, OSU requires all departments to have centralized practice plans. All new university faculty members must join their respective department practice plans. We believe the pediatric faculty practice plan will continue, probably with some modifications, such as contractual relationships with pediatric surgical specialties. The main advantage of the plan is its ability to attract faculty members whose primary focus is academic medicine.

## Organization and Management

PAA is a not-for-profit educational practice plan (501C.3). Its purposes are to:

▲ Provide medical care to all sick and injured children, without regard to ability to pay.

▲ Engage in biomedical research.

▲ Provide clinical and classroom instruction to students enrolled in OSU-COM and to residents and fellows employed at or affiliated with Children's Hospital.

PAA is incorporated with a single shareholder—the chair of the board of directors and of the Department of Pediatrics.

The board of directors of the corporation consists of faculty members of PAA, who are elected (hired) by the sole shareholder of the corporation.

## Governance

The chair has the sole authority to elect (hire) members of the board. The shareholder also determines the salary and compensation packages of all directors. Except for hiring of faculty and establishing faculty compensation, all decisions and actions of PAA are the direct responsibility of the board of directors. It delegates the responsibility of PAA day-to-day operations to an executive committee. The eight-member executive committee consists of four directors elected at large, two directors appointed by the chair, the executive director, and the chair. The executive committee meets weekly, and its actions are approved by the board at quarterly meetings.

## Practice Settings

Practice settings include inpatient units at Children's Hospital, the neonatal intensive care unit at the Ohio State University Medical Center, a pediatric oncology consultation service at the James Cancer Hospital on the OSU campus, a community hospital special care nursery, and pediatric subspecialty consultative services at four community hospitals. In addition, there are several ambulatory practice settings, including the Children's Hospital emergency department and ambulatory clinics, five community ambulatory clinics, and the subspecialty office practices of PAA members. These offices are housed in a single medical office building on the Children's Hospital campus. PAA provides few ancillary services. Radiology, laboratory medicine, and cardiodiagnostic services are provided by Children's Hospital.

## Revenue and Expense Distributions

The corporation accounts for revenue and expense at two levels—corporate and section. The sections are the 22 pediatric subspecialty groups in PAA. Revenues are received from three sources: patient care, contracts with hospitals, and research grant funds. If revenue exceeds expenses at the corporate level, the amount in excess of expenses is split 50 percent to a Chair's Fund and 50 percent to sections that have revenues in excess of expenses. Section funds are divided among sections in proportion to their profitability. The expenses of the less profitable sections are covered by revenues in excess of expenses derived from the profitable sections that are not distributed to the section and by monies from the Chair. The money in the section funds can be used at the discretion of the section for any purpose that furthers patient care or the academic mission of the section. The money cannot, however, be used to increase individual compensation. Section expenses include:

▲ Physician salaries and fringe benefits.

▲ Office and clinic expenses.

▲ Clerical support.

▲ Utilities and miscellaneous costs.

▲ A prorated administrative charge (approximately 15 percent of section revenues).

▲ A tax to the Chair's Fund (10 percent of section revenues).

The Chair's Fund supports the academic functions of the corporation. The chair uses it to support faculty research, new faculty recruitment, faculty travel to national meetings, etc.

## Faculty Compensation

Direct faculty compensation (i.e., salary plus fringe benefits) is set by the PAA board chair. An attempt is made to keep salaries between the 50 and 80 percent of the American Association of Medical Colleges' salary survey.[2] Individual PAA members receive compensation directly from OSU for their teaching and research efforts. The amount of OSU compensation varies among members. The PAA board chair adjusts PAA salary compensation of individual directors to maintain relative equity among faculty members of similar academic rank.

In addition, faculty members may work evening clinics at an hourly rate. This "moonlighting" income is unlimited. Faculty members, according to academic rank, also may earn $3,500 to $5,500 per year in book royalties and honoraria. The faculty incentive for patient care activities is only $0.25 per patient contact.

## Successes

PAA has been successful at accomplishing its primary purposes. There is a single system for seeing all pediatric patients, regardless of their socioeconomic status. More than 50 percent of patients are Medicaid recipients. The growth in patient volume is reflected by an increase in emergency department visits to Children's Hospital from approximately 50,000 to 71,000 per year. The emergency department is the second busiest pediatric emergency department in the United States. PAA captures more than 90 percent of the pediatric subspecialty market in its referral area.

The full-time pediatric faculty of the department of pediatrics has trebled since 1981, when there were 29 faculty members (26 MDs and 3 PhDs). Now there are 105 faculty members (96 MDs and 9 PhDs.) Turnover of faculty members has remained extremely low (1-2 per year). The highest faculty turnover has occurred in the sections of neonatology and emergency medicine. Turnover in these areas may reflect a dissatisfaction with the PAA compensation program.

Success in teaching is reflected by a consistent 100 percent matching of more than 20 pediatric residency positions each year. Teaching evaluations completed by OSU medical students consistently rate the pediatric faculty as among the best of the OSU College of Medicine. *U.S. News & World Report* ranked the OSU College of Medicine as among "America's best" (1992-1994) for primary care medical training.[3]

Research activity at Children's Hospital has increased dramatically since incorporation of PAA. In 1978, total extramural grant support was $638,000, of which $212,000 was received from the National Institutes of Health. In 1992, total extramural support was $6,600,000. Funded NIH grants amounted to $3,600,000.

## Failures

The major failure of PAA was a decrease in financial support from the OSU College of Medicine. Each year, PAA contributed $80,000 to $90,000 to the College of Medicine. Perceived as a thriving department, pediatrics received less in return.

Although the Central Ohio health care market is less than 20 percent managed care, this will change in the near future. The PAA is well positioned for a managed care market. Most faculty salaries are competitive, and none are excessive. The lack of financial incentive for patient care activities, however, may present problems. Currently, physicians are given a token incentive to see patients ($0.25 per encounter). This makes it difficult to convince faculty to take on new clinical duties and to obtain billing information from them. Stronger incentives are being considered, but they have not yet been defined. In addition, PAA has no mechanism to ensure optimum utilization. As the managed care market increases in Central Ohio, utilization management will be an essential program. In addition, development is under way of an integrated delivery system that will involve Children's Hospital, our practice plan, surgical subspecialties, and practicing pediatricians. The already negotiates its own managed care contracts, but also participates in physician hospital organizations.

## References

1. McGarey, M. *Children's Grows up—A Century of Caring.* Columbus, Ohio: Children's Hospital, Inc., 1992, p. 89.

2. Smith, W. *1994-1995 Report on Medical School Faculty Salaries.* Washington, D.C.: Association of American Medical Colleges, 1996.

3. "Graduate Schools." *U.S. News & World Report,* March 23, 1992, March 22, 1993, and March 21, 1994.

*James A. Menke, MD, is Associate Professor of Pediatrics, Richard E. McClead, MD, is Associate Professor, and Mitchell Wheller, BS, MHA, is an Administrator, Department of Pediatrics, Ohio State University, Columbus, Ohio.*

# Chapter 13

▲ ▲ ▲

## Centralization Characterizes University of Arkansas Plan

by F. Patrick Maloney, MD, MPH

## Organizational Structure

Until recently, the Practice Plan at the University of Arkansas School of Medicine was called the Medical College Physicians Group (MCPG), and all full-time faculty in clinical practice were participants in the program. Part-time faculty members could participate by special arrangement. In 1996, the faculty voted to establish a Faculty Group Practice (FGP). Because FGP is still in its developmental phase and the bylaws have not been approved by the Board of Trustees, both MCPG and FGP are described here.

The plan was structured as "an unincorporated division of the College of Medicine" and, as part of the University's Medical Sciences Campus, "is subject to the policies and regulations of the College of Medicine." The University of Arkansas has several campuses, the Medical Sciences Campus being one of them. The organizational chart for MCPG is shown in figure 1, page 100. The chancellor reports to the president and to the board of trustees of the university. FGP accountability is same as that for MCGP. The organizational structure is shown in figure 2, page 100.

## Management

The FGP Executive Committee is responsible for management of FGP. The Executive Committee must "function within the Bylaws, Rules and Regulations of MCPG and must be responsive to the membership of MCPG and accountable for meeting institutional objectives and", at the same time, "be responsive to the University and State laws and regulations, the Dean of the College of Medicine, and the Chancellor of the Campus."*

The MCPG board consisted of:

▲ Chair of each College of Medicine clinical department

▲ Dean, College of Medicine (*ex officio* with vote)

▲ Medical directors of Arkansas Children's Hospital (ACH) and University Hospital (UH)

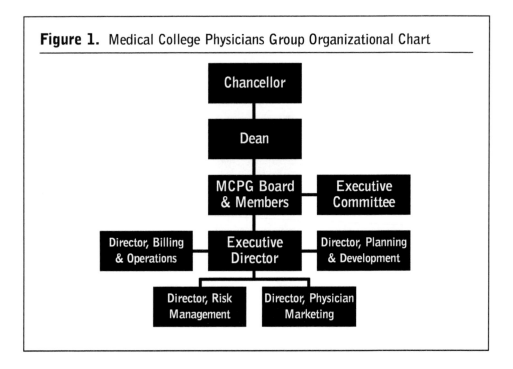

**Figure 1.** Medical College Physicians Group Organizational Chart

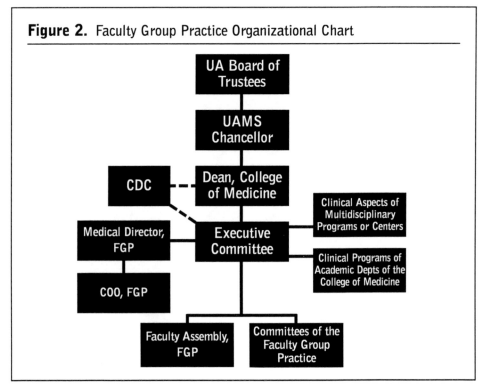

**Figure 2.** Faculty Group Practice Organizational Chart

▲ Executive directors of ACH and UH.

▲ One member-at-large, elected by the membership from the pool of members who primarily practice at UH.

▲ One member-at-large, elected by the membership from the pool of members who primarily practice at ACH and represent pathology, radiology, psychiatry, and anesthesiology.

▲ One member-at-large, elected by the membership from the pool of members who primarily practice at ACH and represent the surgical specialty services.

▲ One additional member from department of medicine, appointed by the chair of the department.

▲ Two additional members from department of pediatrics, appointed by the department chair.

▲ Director, Arkansas Cancer Research Center (ACRC).

▲ ACH division chief, representative of Executive Committee.

▲ Executive Director of MCPG.

▲ All chiefs of independent clinical divisions of the College of Medicine.

The FGP Executive Committee members serve for three-year terms, except for one- and two-year initial terms. The total number of voting members of the committee is 11. The membership of the committee consists of:

▲ The Dean, College of Medicine, *ex officio*, without vote.

▲ The Chief Operating Officer of FGP or his or her equivalent position, *ex officio*, without vote.

▲ The Medical Director of FGP, *ex officio*, without vote.

▲ At least six chairs of clinical departments.

▲ Two primary care physicians.

▲ Three physicians who practice at Arkansas Children's Hospital.

▲ One basic science chair.

▲ At least three nonchairs.

Members are expected to act as representatives of all group practice physicians and practitioners. The Executive Committee has approved the following committees:

▲ Finance and Operations.

▲ Managed Care.

▲ Practice Development.

▲ Professional Standards.

▲ Clinical Research.

MCPG had an Executive Director, a full-time position that required a management background and was responsible for supervision of staff. This person was appointed by the board upon recommendation of the Executive Committee, but required the concurrence of the Dean of the College of Medicine. The equivalent FGP position is a Chief Operating Officer. Other management positions are directors of risk management and physician recruiting, a project coordinator, and other appointments by the Executive Committee.

## Governance
Ultimate governance lies with the University Board of Trustees. In practice, the MCPG board was and the FGP Executive Committee is the functional governing body. However, it has responsibility through the Dean, Chancellor, and President of the university.

## Practice Settings
The main practice setting is at University Hospital and the Medical Sciences Campus. However, members of the faculty also practice off-site at Children's Hospital, at off-site outpatient clinics for family practice and obstetrics/gynecology, and at a rehabilitation hospital. In addition to University Hospital, the campus includes Arkansas Cancer Research Center, Ambulatory Care Center, Jones Eye Center, and family practice clinics. The Veterans Administration Hospital is a two-division hospital with an acute care division adjacent, and physically connected, to University Hospital by a bridge. The chronic care division is located in North Little Rock, about seven miles away. All area hospitals are within a 20-minute or less drive of each other. Several faculty members have consulting privileges at a variety of local hospitals. In addition, faculty members serve at area health education centers (AHECs) at six Arkansas locations, and, more recently, relationships are being established with a network of community health services.

## Revenue and Expense Distributions
Revenue and expenses are centralized with FGP for billing and collection purposes. FGP billing overhead is 10.25 percent of net revenue, and the Dean's Fund is 8 percent. For most departments, an additional 1 percent is collected for program seed money. Income from all sources is deposited in a department professional fees account in campus ledgers. This means that dollars from practice plan billings and from other clinical contractual sources are commingled.

## Faculty Compensation
The practice plans are flexible; different departments may have different plans (figure 3, page 103). The most common plan, Plan A, establishes a base salary and benefits plus a quarterly incentive bonus. The base salary of each faculty member is negotiated annually with the department chair and then with the Dean. It combines state-supported dollars and anticipated professional fee income, based, in part, on the faculty member's financial history. Physician compensation is limited to three times the state-allowed base for full-time faculty for all campuses. A few exceptions are made for highly sought-after and highly paid specialties, such as cardiac surgery and neurosurgery, with the Board of Trustees' approval. The salary goal includes an additional quarterly incentive bonus based on the usual anticipated department income, the anticipated income of the faculty member, the state faculty salary cap limitation, and the finances of the School of Medicine. For example, if the department and faculty member are doing well financially and continuation is anticipated, the base salary

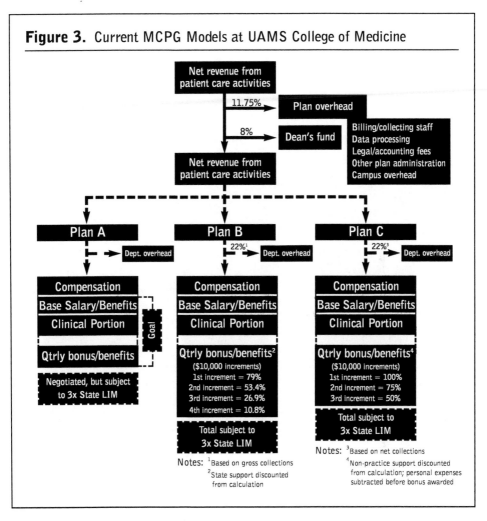

**Figure 3.** Current MCPG Models at UAMS College of Medicine

may be increased. If, on the other hand, finances are problematic, the base salary may not be increased and the increase, if any, is placed in the quarterly bonus. Payment of the bonus always depends on the department's being in a positive financial situation, regardless of whether the individual has a positive cash flow.

A few departments have developed variations of this schema (figure 2). These departments have histories of very positive financial situations. The net or gross earnings are taxed at 22 percent for department overhead, and the remainder is returned to the individual. The amount returned to the individual varies in percentage according to $10,000 increments, as outlined in the figure. For example, in Plan B, 79 percent of the first increment is distributed to the individual and 21 percent to the department. In the second increment, 53.4 percent goes to the individual, etc. In Plan C, 100 percent of the first increment is distributed, 75 percent of the second increment, etc. However, the 22 percent tax to the departments vary, based on gross collections in Plan B and on net collections in Plan C.

Yet another plan (Plan D) has been started that assigns points to a variety of teaching, research/scholarship, and other committee work and permits an accumulation of points that are factored into the incentive plan. This is a rather elaborate schema that has not, thus far, been widely utilized, although it is being encouraged and may emerge as a common plan.

Finally, most nonphysicians in a clinical department, do not participate in the faculty practice plan unless they generate clinical income. The indirect costs of grants are not given back directly to the departments. A portion of indirect costs generated by medical school faculty members are used by the Dean for various department developmental needs. In order to provide incentives to these faculty members, a plan in which a proportion of the dollars attributed to the faculty member's salary on their grants is given back to the faculty member. Fifteen percent is given for the first 25 percent of salary supported by grant, 20 percent for the second 25 percent, and 25 percent for the remainder of the salary or proportion thereof.

## Successes and Failures in This Model

The model is flexible enough to permit the aforementioned variations. There is a high degree of collegiality among the chairs and the division chiefs. Seed money for new initiatives can be funded wholly or in part. A departure from strict university control was a cooperative effort to obtain permission from the Board of Trustees to establish a managed care vehicle independent of the University. This company will have primarily university physicians as core members and will have board control, but will have board members from other sources, will reach all parts of the state, will involve other area hospitals, and will involve volunteer faculty and nonfaculty member primary care panels.

The major problems that have arisen are slowness of reaction time to the changing medical environment, nonuniformity of fees across departments, low number of primary care specialists versus high proportion of specialists, difficulty in a state system in developing a marketing arm of the practice plan, and heavy reliance on inpatient versus outpatient treatments. The heavy emphasis on maximizing clinical income has spawned a new nontenured university track for clinicians within primary care departments and divisions. This heavy emphasis on revenue generation has interfered, to some extent, with some departments' teaching missions. The higher costs of providing care in a university health sciences center become problematic in marketing to managed care providers.

Developments in recent months involve cooperation with the university-generated managed care corporation, consolidation of activities, expansion of outpatient activities, building and remodeling facilities (for example, a new bed tower is being built for University Hospital, four additional floors have been added to the Arkansas Cancer Research Center, and a new eye institute has opened). Uniform fees have been developed, a marketer has been hired by the practice plan, a person to develop and relate to managed care companies has been put in place, and a managed care committee has been established.

Under consideration is the development of Plan D for department practice plans. Distribution of revenues after allocation for department overhead is shown in figure 4, page 105. An incentive component provided according to academic performance as well as clinical performance is based on a rather elaborate point system (figure 5, page 106).

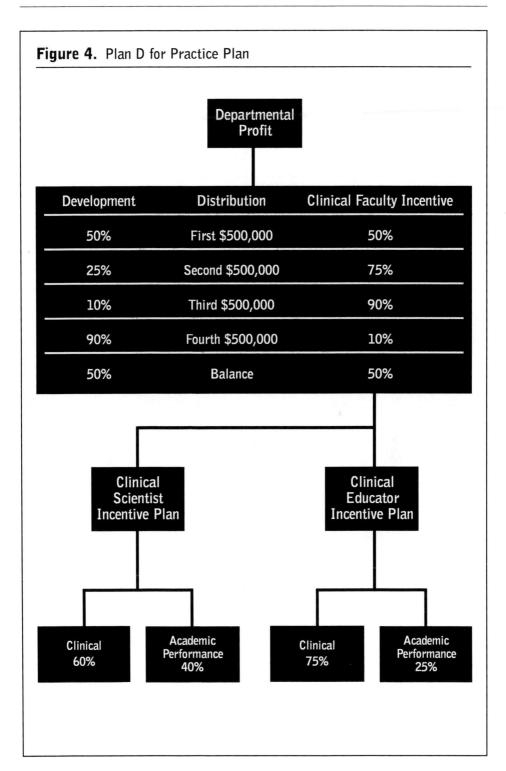

**Figure 4.** Plan D for Practice Plan

**Figure 5.** Point System Used in Plan's Incentive Component

| Goals | Measurements | | 250 |
|---|---|---|---|
| Strong, competitive residency program | Department Senior Elective Student teaching more than 6 month/year | 5 | |
| | Didactic lectures/courses for students/residents | 1 per | |
| Excellence in teaching | Categorical course – head | 5 | |
| | Procedural teaching | 5 | |
| Increased participation in teaching | Organ system teaching | 5 | |
| | Medical Student Teaching Coordinator | 10 | |
| | Residency Training Director | 50 | |
| | Postgraduate Course Director | 5 | |
| | Annual teaching award | 5 | |
| | Summary score on faculty evaluations by resident | 3 for 3, 4 for 4, 5 for 5 | 125 |
| | Summary score on faculty evaluations by students | 3 for 3, 4 for 4, 5 for 5 | points |
| **Research/Scholarship** Strong research project | Scientific exhibits | 3 per exhibit | |
| | Publication in peer-review journals | 4 (1ᵗ/2ⁿ/Sr. author; 2 per) | |
| | Publication in non peer-review journals | 2 | |
| Increase in federally funded research | Paper presentation at peer meeting—specialty society | 4 per | |
| | Paper presentation at peer meeting—RSNA, ARRS | 4 per | |
| | Book chapter | 5 per | |
| Initiatives in new research areas | Book | 10 | |
| | Editorial board/book editor—not journal review done | 3 per | |
| | Grant applications (PI or PI or Project in PPG) | 2 per renewal or new grants | |
| National prominence in specialty area | Grant award (PI or PI or Project in PPG) | 5 per | |
| | Increase in salary support from research activity | 10 per | |
| | Departmental Research Coordinator | 4 (5%); 8 (10%); 12 (15%) | |
| | Visiting Professor | 8 | |
| | Journal Reviewer | 5 per | |
| | Conferences and consultations | 2 per | 125 |
| | Publication of case reports | 1 per | points |
| **Other** | Committee work within Department | 6 (leadership); 4 (member) per | |
| | Committee work within institution | 6 (leadership); 4 (member) per | |
| | Committee work National/State | 6 (leadership); 4 (member) per | |
| | American Board of Specialty Examiner | 5 | |
| | Residency Review Commission | 5 | |
| | Certification of Added Qualifications | 5 | |
| | Officer of National Organization | 10 | |
| | Officer of Local Organization | 3 | |
| | Departmental Division Head | 10 | |
| | Section Head | 8 | |
| | Fellowship Award (one time only) | 5 | |
| | NIH Study Section Reviewer | 10 | |
| | Private/National Reviewer | 10 | |
| | Student Advisor/Resident Mentor | 3 per | 125 |
| | Court Appearance | 2 | points |

A group is currently reviewing the practice plans to develop more specific guidelines and uniformity:

▲ Goals of Faculty Incentive Plan

Equitably promote and distribute proceeds from profitable activity.

Reward and stimulate excellence in performance.

Promote balance of service, research, and academic priorities.

Develop a framework for design and execution of managed care.

Retain and recruit quality faculty.

Encourage teamwork and cohesiveness.

Maintain financial viability of the clinical departments.

▲ Elements of Incentive Plan

Eligibility requirements.

Scoring mechanism/rating factors.

Determination of available income (for distribution).

Data to be used in scoring.

Frequency of incentive plan distribution.

Definition of salary adjustments/criteria not tied to FIP.

▲ Base Salary Equity

Committee recommendation to achieve and maintain 80 percent base, 20 percent incentive ratio

▲ Managed Care Initiatives

Write plans that promote profitability as well as productivity.

— Develop information systems using data obtained from managed care organizations to track physician performance.

— Incorporate physician performance criteria into faculty incentive plan (FIP).

▲ Address (Re)Distribution of State Dollars

Departments may wish to reallocate state dollars to better separate activities that are not directly related to clinical (earned income) endeavors.

▲ Nonsalary Incentives

Books, dues, subscriptions, and travel

— Negotiate nonsalary incentives separately from FIP.

— Establish income distribution to fund faculty development fund and cover nonsalary related expenses

▲ Define Department Overhead Contribution

Departments define distribution of revenue to cover operating expenses and communicate their plans to the faculty.

All department income sources, including but not limited to state appropriations, professional fee income, and external sources such as grant funds, are addressed in the overhead contribution formula.

Revenue distribution addresses the following expense categories:

— Faculty development

— Administrative overhead (operating expense)

— Chairman's discretionary fund

▲ Equity between Tenure Tracks (Academic versus Clinical)

Departments must develop incentive plans that reflect the different tenure track plans but do not penalize one tenure track over the other.

▲ Use of Relative Value Units as Standard Measure of Clinical Performance

\* Constitution and By-laws, University of Arkansas for Medical Sciences, Medical College Physicians Group, Approved by Board of Trustees, 1993.

*F. Patrick Maloney, MD, MPH, is Professor and Chair, Department of Physical Medicine and Rehabilitation, College of Medicine, University of Arkansas for Medical Sciences (UAMS), Little Rock. The author extends appreciation to William C. Hilles, MA, Associate Dean, UAMS College of Medicine, for his helpful information and review of this manuscript.*

# Chapter 14

▲  ▲  ▲

## A Faculty Practice Plan within a Community/University Integrated Medical Education Program

by Tom M. Johnson, MD, FACP, and John L. Jones Jr., MA, MBA

*D*istribution of physician professional fee income among practicing academic physicians is without a doubt the greatest single cause of controversy and organizational dissonance within this group of medical professionals. Practice plans, per se, have long been said to be the great Achilles' heel of medical school deans; many have lost their jobs over physicians professional fee distribution plans.

Michigan State University-Kalamazoo Center for Medical Studies (MSU/KCMS) is a partnership of Michigan State University's College of Human Medicine and two community teaching hospitals. The corporate body of MSU/KCMS is established as a 501c.3 corporation and is a consortium-based, community/university, integrated medical education program. Presently, MSU/KCMS employs more 50 full-time equivalent (FTE) physician faculty members and 135 resident physicians in eight graduate medical education programs. Forty medical students from Michigan State University's College of Human Medicine take their entire clinical training in Kalamazoo.

### Why Develop a Practice Plan?
The MSU/KCMS Board of Directors in 1988 reorganized the corporation in order to meet changing Residency Review Committee requirements. A major focus was to increase the number of full-time employed faculty physicians. Because of the increased number of full-time employed physicians and concerns by the board and practicing community physicians, several options for faculty compensation were considered, from straight salary to some form of incentive for additional practice. The board ultimately decided that administration of the corporation should proceed with the development of a practice plan in order to have control over practice opportunities for employed faculty physicians.

### How the Plan Was Developed
Prior to 1989 and implementation of the practice plan, members of the MSU/KCMS physician faculty were on straight salary. Implementation of a plan in which compensation is at risk was a significant change. MSU/KCMS administrators sought the help of a nationally recognized consultant who managed a large university practice plan. The consultant spent

the first several visits interviewing faculty and board members. Over the next several months, a plan was developed with faculty input. Finally, in early 1990, the plan was presented to the faculty at large and then to the Board.

A key concept of implementation was to run a parallel system for one year. That is, faculty members remained on straight salary for one year but were provided quarterly information throughout the year regarding salary performance as if they were on the plan. After the one-year trial, faculty members were integrated into the plan.

## How the Plan Works

The entire plan document is shown in the appendix to this chapter. Here, however, the compensation component will be described in greater detail.

For this example, we will assume a faculty member has a base salary of $100,000. The base is broken into two components: academic and practice. The exact percentages for the academic and practice components are determined in negotiations between the CEO/Community Dean and the Residency Program Directors. This is a major weakness of the plan, in that the allocations are at best an educated guess.

It is assumed that this faculty member would derive 50 percent of his or her salary for academic duties and 50 percent for practice activities. The faculty member is paid the $100,000 in equal installments throughout the year. In this phase, the corporation assumes up-front risk for practice.

Throughout the academic year, the faculty member is required to earn the practice component plus overhead. The physician is provided quarterly statements and incentive payments if he or she earns in excess of the quarterly practice requirement plus overhead costs.

If we assume the faculty member generated $150,000 through practice activity, the practice component would be calculated as follows:

| | |
|---|---|
| Earned through practice | $150,000 |
| Overhead costs at 50 percent | -75,000 |
| Practice component | -50,000 |
| | |
| Dollars to Incentive Component | $ 25,000 |

The incentive component is paid as follows:

| | |
|---|---|
| 60 percent | $15,000 to physician |
| 30 percent | $ 7,500 to department |
| 10 percent | $ 2,500 to dean |

Further rules were found to be necessary:

▲ The incentive component cannot exceed 125 percent of base. This ensures that the faculty member does not spend to much time in practice, ignoring academic requirements.

▲ If the faculty member meets the practice component plus overhead and the incentive payment is available, the physician always receives his or her incentive component.

▲ The department payment and the dean's payment are made only if all members of a department earn the practice component of the base. If they do not, the dean's and the department components reimburses the corporation for the base salary risk of the practice component.

▲ Overhead is determined on the basis of Medical Group Management Association (MGMA) data for physician groups of similar size. This avoids the necessity for expensive cost accounting systems at the start.

## Analysis

The plan worked well for high-volume and procedure-based specialties, such as family practice, orthopedic surgery, and general surgery. However, making the practice component was difficult for internal medicine, pediatrics, and pediatric subspecialties.

As the plan progressed, faculty became disenchanted with the perceived arbitrary way in which the practice and academic components were derived. Faculty soon discovered that, if the academic component were higher and the practice component lower, their ability to earn an incentive increased proportionately. Some faculty argued this point very vigorously. Such arguments led to a significant disenchantment among faculty members regarding the plan.

Over time, the faculty began to feel that the mechanics of the plan were too complicated, and misunderstandings began to occur. Faculty members became skeptical of the plan and its administration. The plan was administered centrally through the community dean's office. The chief financial officer (CFO) managed the day to day operations. Faculty members expressed great reluctance to have the CFO manage the plan so closely because they perceived that the organization was too financially driven at the expense of academic needs. Also, data presented to faculty were confusing, particularly in terms of complexity related to splits, quarterly statements, overages, and underages. An accuracy question related to the patient billing function arose. Trust between plan administration and physicians became of primary concern.

In early 1994, the board suspended the plan, placed physicians back on straight salary, and instructed administration to develop a new compensation plan for physicians. The reasons for suspending the plan revolved around the general unhappiness of the faculty with the plan. The board asked administration to develop a new faculty compensation plan that considered lessons learned over the previous four to five years. The new CEO/community dean assembled a faculty group, and a new plan was implemented July 1, 1995.

## Analysis, New Plan

Surprisingly, the new plan has worked quite well. The parameters of the plan placed all full-time physicians back to straight salary. Portions of each salary were allocated to the clinical cost center to form a physician salary targeted expense. The amount allocated to clinical cost centers was at least as much as required under the old plan. Instead of individual physicians' being required to hit certain financial parameters, the onus was put on the whole department—for example, family practice. The salary expense target having been worked out, the remainder of the clinical cost center income statement could be constructed with known direct and indirect expenses. At year-end, any excess of revenues over expenses was allocated as follows:

▲ 60 percent to the department research and educational fund.

▲ 30 percent back to the hospital partners.

▲ 10 percent to the assistant dean research and educational fund.

What was surprising to us is that, if given fair compensation, academic faculty members have the incentive to achieve financial targets and control clinical costs to further support their teaching and research missions through research and education funds. These funds are under the control of the department chair and can be used for travel, fellowships, additional faculty, resident conference, etc. The funds cannot be used for salary. The CEO/community dean conducted a study prior to implementing this plan to understand teaching time versus practice time. Having this information allowed him to fairly set practice parameters. We are comfortable that practice is not the driving force over education. Yet we are also comfortable with the fact that adequate funds are being derived from practice to support the educational mission of the consortium.

# Appendix

## Michigan State University
## Kalamazoo Center For Medical Studies
## Faculty Practice Plan

## Preamble

The Kalamazoo community, Michigan State University Kalamazoo Center for Medical Studies, Inc. (MSU/KCMS), its Members, and its full-time faculty will benefit from the establishment of a faculty practice plan (hereinafter referred to as the "Plan"). While the Plan is developed for full-time, regular faculty of MSU/KCMS whose professional activities in teaching, research, and patient care are conducted as part of the Plan, professional services provided by volunteer faculty members on behalf of MSU/KCMS are recognized as vital to the success of the Plan and MSU/KCMS.

The primary goal of the MSU/KCMS Faculty Practice Plan is to diversify the financial base of MSU/KCMS through the generation of institutional and programmatic fund support in order to:

1. Attract, retain, and reward high-quality, full-time faculty through the establishment of a mechanism that recognizes and supports excellence in graduate medical education, medical research, and patient care activity.

2. Augment the ability of the Kalamazoo medical community to attract and support new specialists and subspecialist physicians.

## Article I
## Establishment of a Faculty Practice Plan

**Section 1.01. Name.** The name of the faculty practice plan established under the auspices of the By-laws of Michigan State University Kalamazoo Center for Medical Studies will be entitled "Michigan State University Kalamazoo Center for Medical Studies Faculty Practice Plan."

**Section 1.02. Faculty Practice Plan Policies.** All policies, rules, and procedures as contained in this document and all rules, procedures, and practices derived from the document will conform with the By-laws of the Corporation, and its established policies, rules, procedures, and practices.

**Section 1.03. Authorization.** The MSU/KCMS Faculty Practice Plan is incorporated into and authorized by the Bylaws of the Corporation.

**Section 1.04. Terms.** The definition of terms to be used by the Plan will be as follows:

A. *MSU/KCMS:* Michigan State University Kalamazoo Center for Medical Studies, the Corporation under which the Plan will be organized.

B. *Corporation:* The legal nonprofit entity, established under the rules of the State of Michigan, that is the corporate body of MSU/KCMS.

C. *Corporate Members:* The legal members to the partnership that established MSU/KCMS, including: Michigan State University College of Human Medicine, Borgess Medical Center, and Bronson Methodist Hospital.

D. *Board of Directors:* The Board of MSU/KCMS.

E. *Executive Committee:* The standing committee of the MSU/KCMS Board of Directors established by the By-laws of the Corporation.

F. *Finance Committee:* The standing committee of the MSU/KCMS Board of Directors that oversees all financial aspects of the Corporation.

G. *President/CEO:* The primary officer of the Corporation who serves as a Member of the Board of Directors and concurrently serves as the Assistant Dean for MSU College of Human Medicine.

H. *Plan Member:* All full-time, nontenured track faculty members who are employed by MSU/KCMS and who are designated to participate in the Plan.

I. *Income:* Any financial remuneration that is received by Members of the Plan.

J. *Overhead:* Any and all costs associated with the organization and the implementation of all programs under the auspices of MSU/KCMS.

K. *Faculty Practice Plan Advisory Committee:* The committee with oversight responsibility for the activities of the MSU/KCMS Faculty Practice Plan.

L. *Department:* The organizational unit that defines all clinical programs at MSU/KCMS.

## Article II
## Purpose

**Section 2.01. Purpose.** The Plan will delineate policies and procedures that relate to the operation and use of all income generated by the faculty of MSU/KCMS to meet the goals of the Plan and MSU/KCMS.

A. To specify procedures by which faculty practice plan income will be managed to supplement basic support of programs.

B. To sustain and enhance faculty incentives to engage in MSU/KCMS programs.

C. To generate institutional funds for the purposes of recruiting and retaining qualified faculty necessary to develop and sustain MSU/KCMS programs in medical research and graduate medical education.

D. To act as an institutional agent for innovation in educational programs and health care delivery.

## Article III
## Plan Member

**Section 3.01. Membership.** A Plan Member is a physician licensed in the State of Michigan or a licensed health care professional holding a full-time, nontenured track faculty position with MSU College of Human Medicine who is employed at MSU/KCMS. A Plan Member will conduct all of his or her professional teaching, research, and clinical care activities as part of the Plan.

**Section 3.02. Outside Activities.** A Plan Member will not engage in the private practice of medicine except in keeping with the policies of MSU/KCMS, waives any right to receive direct compensation from other than MSU/KCMS for health care service of any nature, and assigns all rights to such compensation to MSU/KCMS.

## Article IV
## Plan Income

**Section 4.01. Definition.** For purposes of the Plan, plan income refers to and includes all bills arising from the diagnosis, treatment, and care of patients generated by full-time, non-tenured faculty members and resident-supervised activities of the Department regardless of location of service and as part of their MSU/KCMS assigned responsibilities.

**Section 4.02. Other Income Sources.** Other compensation sources as approved by the MSU/KCMS Executive Committee may be considered Plan income.

**Section 4.03. Income Excluded from the Plan.** Income excluded from the Plan is that income generated by a Plan Member that is nonclinical in nature. Specific types of income that are excluded include:

A. Royalties

B. Honoraria

C. Administrative consulting fees

D. Speaking fees

E. Investment income

**Section 4.04. Time Allowed for Outside Income Generation.** While the generation of outside income is allowed by the Plan, it is anticipated that time spent in generating outside income will not interfere with the contractual objectives of the Plan Member's full-time responsibilities at MSU/KCMS. The Assistant Dean and President/CEO of MSU/KCMS maintains oversight authority for the time commitment of all Plan Members and faculty of MSU/KCMS.

# Article V
# Compensation

**Section 5.01. Total Compensation.** A Plan Member's total compensation including incentives will be determined by a Compensation Committee consisting of the Assistant Dean and President/CEO and a representative appointed by each of the MSU/KCMS Corporate Members.

**Section 5.02. Overhead Expenses.** Overhead expenses will include an administrative component and/or a clinical component. The percentages used for purposes of allocation under the plan will utilize the average of such costs derived from the most recent data sources available from the Health Care Financing Administration (HCFA) or Medical Group Management Association (MGMA). The Faculty Practice Plan Advisory Committee will review the existing overhead policy of the Faculty Practice Plan by the end of March each year. The Faculty Practice Plan Administrator will present a review of MGMA data and other sources of overhead rates by February each year to assist the Faculty Practice Plan Advisory Committee. A recommendation will be made to the Assistant Dean and President/CEO and subsequently to the corporation's Board of Directors on the proposed overhead rate for the next fiscal year.

**Section 5.03. Components of the Plan.** Each Plan Member will have the opportunity to receive a base component and an incentive component. The definition of each component is as follows:

A. Base Component: The base component is provided to the Member for the purposes of teaching, administrative activities related to the organization, research, other contracted activities, and patient care responsibilities. The sources of revenue for the base component can be derived from the following sources: a) funds provided by the organization, b) clinical funds, c) research activities, and d) other contracted sources.

B. Incentive Component: The incentive component will consist of all revenue over and above the base component after overhead expenses up to a maximum of 125 percent of the base component. Contributions to the incentive component will be according to the following formula:

   (1) 60% to the Plan Member.

   (2) 30% to a Departmental fund to be used for funding Departmental research and education expenses.

   (3) 10% to the Assistant Dean fund to be used for funding of general programs of the organization.

C. Excess Revenue: The excess revenue above 125% of the base component that is generated by a Member will be disbursed according to the following formula:

   (1) 60% to the Department.

   (2) 40% to the Assistant Dean fund.

**Section 5.04. Departmental Incentive Compensation.** Plan Members may receive a departmental incentive component for nonfinancial contributions to the success of the Department or Corporation programs. The departmental incentive component will not exceed 10% of the Plan Member's base component.

**Section 5.05 Termination of Employment.** In the event a Plan Member terminates employment with MSU/KCMS for any reason, collected outstanding accounts receivable directly attributed to the professional services of the said Plan Member will be paid to the Plan Member on a quarterly basis following the termination for a maximum period of up to six (6) months. Accounts receivable attributable to the Plan Member that are collected after the six (6) month period will accrue to the general fund of the Corporation. The President/CEO will be responsible for preparing a report on such disbursements for review by the Executive Committee.

**Section 5.06 Community Physician Contractual Relationships.** From time to time, MSU/KCMS departments may contract with community physicians on a part-time basis for education, clinical, research, and administrative services. MSU/KCMS will bill and collect for professional fee income derived by such part-time physicians. MSU/KCMS will apply the standard clinical overhead charge to all professional income derived for the services of such contracted physicians. Any deficits related to contractual arrangements will then be allocated to organizational funds. After overhead and deficits are covered, an allocation of 60 percent will be made to the department's fund and 40 percent to the Dean's Fund.

## Article VI
## Organization and Management of the Plan

**Section 6.01. Administrative Responsibility.** Overall administrative responsibility of the Plan shall be vested in the MSU/KCMS Assistant Dean and President/CEO. The Plan will be operated using sound management practices and cost accounting principles. The Vice President of Finance will serve as the administrator of the Faculty Practice Plan under the supervision of the Assistant Dean and President/CEO.

**Section 6.02. Plan Operations.** Direct administration of the day-to-day operations of the Plan may be delegated by the MSU/KCMS Assistant Dean and President/CEO to MSU/KCMS employees and faculty as appropriate.

**Section 6.03. Faculty Practice Plan Committee.** A Faculty Practice Plan Committee will review and recommend all policy related to the Faculty Practice Plan and advise the Assistant Dean and President/CEO on all matters relating to the operation and administration of the Plan. The Committee will meet at least quarterly to conduct the business of the Faculty Practice Plan. All Members of the Plan will have the right to submit written policy changes for consideration by the Faculty Practice Plan Committee.

**Section 6.04. Composition of the Committee.** Members of the Faculty Practice Plan Committee will consist of the Assistant Dean and President/CEO and Residency Program Directors. The Committee will annually elect a chair to serve for a one-year term and up to three consecutive terms.

**Section 6.05. Annual Meeting.** An annual meeting will be held and will be open to all Members of the Faculty Practice Plan. The time and location of such a meeting will be sent to all Members at least two weeks prior to the annual meeting.

**Section 6.06. Final Authority over the Plan.** The Executive Committee of the MSU/KCMS Board of Directors will review the overall operations and finances of the Plan and act on policy recommendations of the Faculty Practice Plan Committee relative to the Plan.

---

*Tom M. Johnson, MD, FACP, is Assistant Dean and Chief Executive Officer and John L. Jones Jr., MA, MBA, is Chief Operating Officer, Michigan State University-Kalamazoo Center for Medical Studies, Kalamazoo.*